Forensic
Occupational
Therapy

Edited by

LORNA COULDRICK MSc, SROT, CertEd, BACP
East Sussex County Council

and

DEBORAH ALRED DipCOT, SROT
East Sussex County Healthcare NHS Trust

W
WHURR PUBLISHERS
LONDON AND PHILADELPHIA

© 2003 Whurr Publishers Ltd
First published 2003
by Whurr Publishers Ltd
19b Compton Terrace
London N1 2UN England and
325 Chestnut Street, Philadelphia PA 19106 USA

Reprinted 2004

British Library Cataloguing in Publication Data

A catalogue record for this book
is available from the British Library.

ISBN 1 86156 367 1

Typeset by Adrian McLaughlin, a@microguides.net

Contents

Acknowledgements

We are immensely grateful to the Specialist Secure Services Team at East Sussex County Healthcare NHS Trust for supporting the development of this book by providing both specialist advice and practical assistance.

We also wish to thank Chas and Tim for providing unwavering support and encouragement throughout.

Contributors

Deborah Alred DipCOT, SROT Debbie is head occupational therapist and clinical governance lead for the Special Secure Services at East Sussex County NHS Trust. This includes Ashen Hill, a 20-bed medium secure unit; Southview, a 20-bed low secure unit and Rosslyn, a rehabilitation hostel for four people. She has experience in various mental health settings including in-patient acute services, day hospital care, rehabilitation and psychiatry of old age both in the NHS and independent sector. She has worked in secure services for seven years and has an interest in issues related to substance misuse and multidisciplinary working. She is undertaking a Masters degree in Occupational Therapy and Management.

Joe Ayres BSc Hons, SROT, PG DipFMH, FETC Joe is head occupational therapist for the male admissions service, high dependency and crisis intervention units in Broadmoor Hospital, part of West London Mental Health NHS Trust. Joe began at Broadmoor as an occupations assistant, later becoming a technical instructor. He completed an in-service degree and holds a postgraduate diploma in Forensic Mental Health. He has worked as an occupational therapist in high secure services for five years and has an interest in assessment, risk management and personality disorders. He is currently undertaking a Masters degree in Mental Health Studies.

Claire Barton DipCOT, SROT Claire works as clinical team leader for Birchwood pre-discharge service at the Bracton Centre, part of Oxleas NHS Trust. She has worked in adult mental health in both elderly and forensic services. Her forensic experience spans nine years between two medium secure units and a hostel. She has developed a particular interest in the Model of Human Occupation and utilized many of its assessments. She is an advocate of the model, having found it especially helpful in involving patients in the planning of their care and in defining and communicating the role of occupational therapy to both the patient and the multiprofessional team.

John Chacksfield DipCOT, SROT John has spent the greater part of his career working in forensic mental health, primarily in a high secure setting but also in medium secure settings. He is also a visiting lecturer and holds a postgraduate certificate in the education of health professionals. Currently, he is a manager in the independent sector (Psycare), running a 10-bed hostel for the rehabilitation of mentally disordered offenders and others with complex needs. His primary interest is in substance misuse among mentally disordered offenders. This interest developed during his work on the forensic addictive behaviours unit at Broadmoor Hospital.

Channine Clarke MSc, SROT Channine has been working in various mental health services since 1990 and qualified, with a first-class honours degree, in 1998. She was seconded to the College of Occupational Therapists for a year, where she helped develop their clinical audit database, provided clinical governance and audit training for therapists around the country, and was one of the primary authors of the *Outcome Measures Information Pack* published in 2001. She is now a senior occupational therapist, co-managing Rosslyn House, a forensic hostel that focuses on community rehabilitation and reintegration.

Lorna Couldrick MSc, SROT, CertEd, BACP Lorna's career has spanned acute and community care, gerontology, social services, mental health and pre- and post-registration education. She established occupational therapy at the newly opened medium secure unit Ashen Hill in 1986 and enjoyed over eight years in forensic services. Seconded to the Health Advisory Service, she assisted in a review of the services provided by Ashworth Hospital. She is also an accredited counsellor with the British Association of Counselling and Psychotherapy and has undertaken training in forensic psychotherapy. She is currently undertaking a PhD. Her research area is sexual expression, disability and professional practice.

Edward Duncan BSc Hons, DipCBP, SROT Edward is a Senior I Occupational Therapist at the State Hospital, Carstairs, Scotland, where he has worked since 1997. Prior to this, his formative experience was as an occupational therapist in community mental health in Glasgow. Edward is also an accredited cognitive behavioural psychotherapist. Edward's primary interest lies in the development of the evidence base within psychosocial mental health interventions – specifically within forensic care. He has a special interest in working with mentally disordered sexual offenders, an area that has formed a central part of his current PhD studies.

Kathryn Harris BSc Hons, SROT Kathryn previously worked in acute in-patient adult mental health services and a psychodynamically orientated day hospital. She moved into forensic services in 1997 working at the Trevor Gibbens Unit, Maidstone, a medium secure service serving the county of Kent. Initially, her remit was to develop the occupational therapy service on the acute admissions ward. Although originally it was a small 15-bed unit, a major expansion programme is now underway including a dedicated 10-bed women's service. Kathryn is part of the development team. She is a member of the multidisciplinary working group for women service users in forensic psychiatry.

Rebecca Hills MSc, DipCOT, SROT Rebecca is now the lead occupational therapist for Westminster, part of Central and North West London Mental Health NHS Trust. At the time of writing, she was head occupational therapist at the Dene, an independent sector unit run by Partnerships in Care. Her Masters degree was in Interprofessional Health and Welfare Studies. Rebecca has worked in a number of medium and low secure services over the past 12 years. While head occupational therapist at Reaside, she managed the occupational therapy service into HMP Birmingham and HMP Brockhill. Again as head occupational therapist at the Bracton Centre, she supervised occupational therapy services for, and worked in, HMP Belmarsh.

Helena Holford DipCOT, SROT Helena is presently the senior occupational therapist at the Three Bridges, a medium secure service which is part of Ealing, Hammersmith and Fulham NHS Trust. She has also worked at Evenlode, a 10-bed medium secure learning disabilities unit in Oxford. Her forensic experience includes both acute and rehabilitation settings. She is interested in the use of the Model of Human Occupation in forensic settings and utilizes many of its assessments in her work. She uses both group and individual interventions and is interested in facilitating good multidisciplinary teamwork.

Catherine Joe DipCOT, SROT, CertMS Catherine has worked in forensic mental health for five years and is currently the head occupational therapist for Forensic Mental Health Services, South West London and St. George's NHS Mental Health Trust. The service has 71 in-patient beds (56 medium secure, 15 minimum secure), community teams, an outpatient sexual offender service and an outpatient post-traumatic stress disorder service. Catherine has worked in the areas of rehabilitation, acute admissions, community mental health teams and eating disorders. Specific interest areas include user involvement and vocational rehabilitation within medium secure settings.

Rebecca Kelly BSc, DipCOT, SROT Rebecca is currently the forensic head occupational therapist for the Oxfordshire Regional Forensic Service consisting of medium, low secure and planned pre-discharge beds. She has an honours degree in Health Care Studies. She has considerable experience in facilitating cognitive behavioural groups and has published an anger-control training manual for practitioners, based on her own experience of running in- and outpatient programmes. She has been working as an occupational therapist in the NHS since 1987 in both inpatient and community adult mental health services and, for the past 13 years, in a medium secure environment.

Marion Martin MA, BA, SROT Marion is a senior lecturer in occupational therapy at the University of Brighton. As well as being a qualified occupational therapist, she has a degree in Psychology and a Masters in Education. For many years, she worked in mental health services and has a special interest in forensic work. She is currently undertaking a PhD on the subject of boredom, which is little understood, despite being universally recognized. It has direct relevance to forensic occupational therapy, as there do appear to be links between boredom, alienation and offending behaviour.

Ann McQue DipCOT, SROT At the time of writing Ann was head occupational therapist for a community forensic mental health team in West Surrey. Her forensic experience includes 16 years in the high secure setting of Broadmoor Hospital. She was first employed as a technical instructor and then, following in-service training, as an occupational therapist. From there she moved to Oak Trees, a medium/low secure unit for three years. For the past two years, she has been enjoying the opportunity of helping patients settle back into the community. She is now head of occupational therapy at the Dene, a 48-bed medium secure service for women. She has particular interest in risk management and community skills.

Phil Morgan BA Hons, SROT At the time of writing, Phil and Mark Spybey were working together in the Continuing Assessment and Support Unit, a 30-bed low secure, forensic rehabilitation service, part of the East London and City Mental Health Trust. Prior to this, Phil worked at the sister unit, the John Howard Centre, which provides a 68-bed, medium secure service. His degree was in Philosophy and Irish Studies. His interests are in the treatment of addictive behaviours and forensic learning disability.

Andrea Neeson BSc Hons, SROT Andrea has worked in a variety of settings since qualifying, and her experience spans both physical and mental health. As a forensic occupational therapist, she has worked for over four years in secure environments. Her first forensic post was in a 15-bed psychiatric intensive care unit, now known as the Rotherfield Unit. At the time of writing, she was in a 30-bed medium secure unit, the Oxford Clinic, at Fairmile Hospital, part of the Oxfordshire Regional Forensic Service. Andrea has now taken on a new challenge and is presently working with individuals with spinal cord injuries.

Rachel Prentice DipCOT, SROT Rachel is head occupational therapist for the Devon and Cornwall Forensic Psychiatric Service, incorporating a learning disability open unit, open-lockable unit for those with enduring mental illness and a medium secure mental health unit. Rachel's interest in forensic occupational therapy began when, as a basic grade in an acute psychiatric ward, she received specialist supervision for two in-patients with forensic histories. She has worked within forensic settings since 1995. Her experience spans admission, rehabilitation, pre- and post-discharge follow-up services. She has held various posts including two as head of department and continues to maintain clinical contact through group and individual work.

Mark Spybey SROT Graduating in 1983, Mark has worked in England and Canada in various psychiatric settings (including hospital and community). He has worked in low and medium secure forensic settings and worked with Phil Morgan in London. He is currently employed as head occupational therapist in Adult Forensic Psychiatry in Newcastle-upon-Tyne. Mark is particularly interested in developing multidisciplinary strategies to enhance the quality of the rehabilitative aspects of forensic care services. He has extensive experience of using the Model of Human Occupation in addition to the recovery model of psychiatric rehabilitation.

Gill Urquhart DipCOT, SROT Gill is currently the head of occupational therapy at the State Hospital's Board For Scotland, and she set up their service in 1997. Prior to this, Gill worked in a variety of management and clinical settings, although adult mental health has always been her preferred area of clinical interest. Gill's interests now are to explore the wider opportunities for occupational therapy within the Forensic Clinical Network in Scotland by forging strong practice links between differing levels of security.

Michelle Walsh MSc, DipCOT, SROT Michelle has worked in medium and high secure services for over 11 years in various acute and rehabilitation settings. She is presently head occupational therapist for women's services at Broadmoor Hospital and manages a unit providing specialist occupational therapy services to women on the high-dependency, crisis-intervention and admission-assessment wards. Michelle's interests include issues relating to self-harm and general mental health services for women. She has pioneered self-harm support groups for women in Broadmoor Hospital and, as part of her Masters in Mental Health, she explored contagion factors in self-harming behaviours. Michelle has also undertaken training in Critical Incident Stress Debriefing.

Kirsty Wilson BSc Hons, SROT Kirsty's first appointment in forensic services was over four years ago when she worked at Leander, a learning disability open unit. Following this, she developed an occupational therapy service for Avon House, a newly commissioned unit for those with enduring mental illness. She is presently Senior I Occupational Therapist at Langdon Hospital, Devon and Cornwall Forensic Psychiatric Service, and is currently responsible for the development and coordination of the vocational rehabilitation service, which is accessed by clients from medium secure and learning disability units. She is particularly interested in multidisciplinary team working and pre-registration education.

Foreword

Since 1990, the demand for occupational therapists to work with mentally disordered offenders and others detained in secure settings has increased dramatically. Although occupational therapists have always been considered essential members of a multidisciplinary team within medium and low secure mental health settings, the recognition of their contribution to assessment and rehabilitation in high security hospitals and prisons is a more recent development. As I know from experience, introducing, managing and developing occupational therapy services provides challenges for both clinicians and managers. This involves negotiating roles, responsibilities, priorities and approaches with staff teams and with the wider organization. The position has been reached where there is also an increasing number of occupational therapists working in forensic settings outside the health sector in the criminal justice service, prisons and the probation service.

From my own practice I know that all these environments present unique challenges to personal and professional beliefs, assumptions and ways of working. If these are not acknowledged and support systems established, the experience of working in forensic services can be punishing and destructive. On a daily basis, forensic occupational therapists experience the tensions of working within the different cultures, norms and expectations that lie at the very interface of the criminal justice and healthcare systems. They have to ensure a secure and safe environment that also has a rehabilitative and risk taking approach both for the individual and the organization without losing sight of public safety. These contradictions and challenges apply at all levels of secure care as well as in the community.

This book highlights the importance of understanding the culture, with its frictions. There are many personal tensions to understand and resolve. These include establishing and maintaining boundaries, coping with security routines, participating in training on the management of aggression, using methods of physical restraint and of working with men and women who have committed offences that the practitioner finds distressing. A common challenge is that of working with people who are detained without length of time and see little point in participating in any activity designed to improve functional abilities. In addition, forensic occupational therapists have to decide how to describe their work in social settings. For example, it is important to learn how to deal with the frequently and strongly expressed views of family, friends, many members of the public and the media that "such people" are not worthy of our professional efforts and expertise.

On the other hand, in forensic services, occupational therapists can practise from a truly holistic perspective and can implement comprehensive and thorough intervention programmes. We have now reached a stage where forensic occupational therapy appears an attractive area of work for students, support staff and practitioners. While this may have made recruitment easier, it has not necessarily improved retention of staff. Reaching a position where our multidisciplinary team colleagues understand our role, support it, challenge it constructively, wish to learn from and with us and share skills, takes confidence, hard work and the ability to look at the whole system in which one operates. This book shares the expertise of many occupational therapists that have considerable experience in forensic work. They all highlight the value they place on using activity as the basis of their intervention. They emphasise the skills required to do so effectively. Most indicate that the use of activity is not the sole preserve of the occupational therapist nor is it the only skill he or she has to offer. If occupational therapists are to feel comfortable in sharing skills and in relinquishing some of the traditional aspects of their work, in order to take on an extended role, they need to do so from a position of confidence in their own role and skills. This book will assist both occupational therapists and other forensic practitioners to clarify and affirm that role. Anyone wishing to work in forensic settings as a practitioner or manager will gain many useful insights from reading this book. For those already working in this area, it will provide the opportunity for reflection and development.

Mary Crawford
NZ Dip OT, SROT, DMS, MIHM

Mary Crawford is the registrant occupational therapist on the Health Professions Council and Chair of the Health Committee on the Health Professions Council. Formerly she was Director of Rehabilitation and Director of Clinical Support Services at Broadmoor Hospital and a consultant to the High Security Psychiatric Services Commissioning Board.

PART ONE
CURRENT PERSPECTIVES

CHAPTER 1
A starting point

LORNA COULDRICK AND DEBORAH ALRED

Introduction

We began the job of editing this book with a mixture of enthusiasm, trepidation and some naivety. We knew from our experience that working with mentally disordered offenders is rewarding, exciting and challenging, but it is also particularly demanding. This can be especially so for occupational therapists, as they belong both to an emerging profession and a minority group in the secure environment (College of Occupational Therapists 1998). Until now there has been a dearth of literature to support practice. This book is written by forensic occupational therapists in the United Kingdom. It describes their experience.

We had a clear view of the literature that we had found useful to our practice as busy therapists. We wanted this to be a book that was easy to read, one that could be enjoyed in a quiet time in the office but which would also inform and stimulate discussion, practice and further reading. We wanted it to be a book based in everyday practice, reflecting some of the complex issues that arise in forensic services, which the reader could relate to. These concepts laid the foundations of our vision.

As our starting point, we contacted occupational therapists working in forensic psychiatry. No specific method was used in choosing authors other than to circulate a draft framework with some guidelines, and the authors' willingness to volunteer. In the process of working on the book a change occurred in the language used. That is, from talking about occupational therapists working in forensic psychiatry to talking with, and writing about, forensic occupational therapists, which is acknowledged in the title of the book.

This chapter provides a profile of the forensic occupational therapist, the rationale for the book, and describes the task we set the authors. The framework of the book is outlined and recurring themes highlighted. This chapter also draws the reader's attention to professional networks, and

1

we hope it gives a flavour of the rewards of working in forensic services. As with all books, it provides a snapshot in time, so this chapter concludes by looking into the future. Some of our omissions are noted, to be addressed by others in future books. The changing context of practice, particularly legislative, is indicated and the need to develop a research culture considered.

Profile of the forensic occupational therapist

Research conducted by the College of Occupational Therapists (Crawford 1998) suggests that the significant majority of occupational therapists working in secure settings have less than three years' experience in forensic psychiatry. Staff employed in support roles as technical instructors and helpers, in the survey, had greater experience especially in the special hospitals. Additionally, many occupational therapists in secure settings work in considerable professional isolation. The majority are employed at Senior I grades, allowing little opportunity to learn their forensic skills under direct professional supervision. This research also highlighted that there was often little occupational therapy input to the strategic planning of services.

Rationale for the book

Added to this limited experience in forensic psychiatry, there is also a paucity of literature to support new occupational therapists embarking on a career within forensic services. Although several books have been published specifically for other professions, particularly nurses, only one such text exists for occupational therapists (Lloyd 1995). Chris Lloyd is an occupational therapist who has worked in forensic services both in Australia and Canada. Her book *Forensic Psychiatry for Health Professionals* provides a well-researched look at the development and delivery of rehabilitation for forensic clients. Its focus is the 'how to' of professional practice. We believe this book complements her work, as it includes recent developments in tools and models and emphasizes the 'what' and 'why' of professional practice. As so little has been written describing forensic occupational therapy, we wanted this book to provide a baseline, a building block, conveying the daily experience of practice.

It could be argued that information on occupational therapy practice should be integrated into an interdisciplinary book on forensic services. Sadly, the main observation of other books is the absence or omission of reference to occupational therapy (Stone et al. 2000, Mercer et al. 2000, Robinson and Kettles 2000, Webb and Harris 1999, Vaughan and Badger 1995). Also, as editors and practitioners, we felt that occupational therapists needed something specifically to support their practice. It is in recognizing and valuing the profession's contribution that confidence is established to work in truly interprofessional ways.

Within the profession, the primary audience for this book is forensic personnel, including support staff and students. However, like a stone thrown into a pond, ripples of the experience, knowledge and expertise, described here, will lap outwards to occupational therapy staff in other settings. This book will be of value to those working in general mental health, long-term residential settings, day care, pre- and post-registration students and, at the outer ripples, even to physical and local authority occupational therapists. Despite totally different contexts of practice, many occupational therapist find themselves working with people who have a personality disorder or forensic history.

Outside the profession, it will be relevant to anyone involved with the planning and development of activity who wants to ensure that this activity is intentionally therapeutic. Other forensic team members will also find something of interest. This book offers an increased understanding of what the occupational therapist is trying to achieve and therefore helps to define where professional roles overlap and complement each other. It is a book about practice in the United Kingdom; nevertheless, we hope it may appeal to an international audience.

The authors' task

The task we set each author was to write about his or her experience, giving everyday examples of issues and cases they encountered. We wanted the book to be grounded in their practice. We told them that our aim was not to produce a heavy, theoretical tome. Rather we hoped each chapter would zing with a sense that this person knows what it is like to work in a forensic setting. In writing, they were not expected to provide all the answers, merely to highlight some of the issues forensic occupational therapists face. Any theory, we said, should be focused on its application to forensic occupational therapy. We did not ask them to include all the scientific and theoretical knowledge in the area, but to signpost further information for readers.

Focus on their experience they did. Each chapter must be read in that knowledge. For example, we have not attempted to make language uniform. Thus, different authors talk of patients, prisoners, clients, residents, offenders and service users. Other terminology, such as task, activity and occupation, or interdisciplinary or multidisciplinary, may have subtly different meanings to each author. For example, John Chacksfield provides a definition of dual diagnosis as mental health and substance misuse, whereas others have used dual diagnosis to indicate a combined diagnosis of mental health and learning disability or personality disorder.

Similarly, some authors work in large regional units where patient numbers mean group work is consistently viable. Others are in small units where group work is impractical. In the same way, all but two chapters are set in England. We have no chapters from practitioners in Wales or Northern Ireland, but the chapters 'Setting up a service' and 'Occupational therapy and the sexual offender' are based on experience in Scotland. The differences in legislation are for the reader to determine.

The framework of the book

Part one of the book, 'Current Perspectives', is intended to provide a context to frame the practice chapters. 'So what is forensic occupational therapy?' by Lorna Couldrick attempts to define the role and clarify why being busy is not, of its own, therapeutic. We believe 'The foundation of good practice' by Marion Martin is a crucial chapter, having observed first-hand forensic occupational therapy floundering due to a mismatch between underpinning theories. So often units do not openly own or describe their theoretical principles; however, nowhere is it more evident that these principles exist than in secure environments.

The majority of forensic occupational therapists work in medium secure settings, so part two takes the reader through 'The occupational therapy process within a medium secure unit'. 'Assessment', written by Claire Barton, is very much a therapist's workbook, which will be particularly helpful for those new to forensic. Other professionals may also find it useful to see the different focus of the occupational therapist's assessment and how that contributes to the interdisciplinary care plan. Throughout the book, authors write about the importance of individual treatment programmes. However, the occupational therapist also has to manage all these individual programmes as a whole. The sum of individual programmes constitutes the unit's programme. Deborah Alred has offered some suggestions for balancing these tensions in 'Programme planning'. 'Everyone is an artist', by Mark Spybey and Phil Morgan, explores the use of creative media in a forensic setting. This and the following chapter, 'Cognitive behavioural group work within forensic occupational therapy', by Rebecca Kelly, demonstrate a little of the vast and varied repertoire of interventions undertaken. Channine Clarke concludes this section with a detailed look at evaluation, in 'Evaluation of forensic occupational therapy practice', again considering evaluation of the occupational therapy programme for the resident and, in terms of clinical governance, for the service.

In part three, we read about the similarities and differences of 'Forensic Occupational Therapy in Other Settings'. Michelle Walsh and Joe Ayres provide a window into 'Occupational therapy in a high-security hospital'.

This chapter also gives a rich history that still has echoes, and implications, for the long-timer being transferred to medium security after perhaps 30 years in Broadmoor. The emerging role of 'The occupational therapist working in prison' is described by Rebecca Hills. She indicates the development of prison healthcare services and the evolving approaches to occupational therapy. Catherine Joe in 'The development of community forensic occupational therapy' has focused on moving from the medical model of disability to a social model. She reminds readers of the need to look at the wider barriers to inclusion. The medical model focuses on improving the skills of the client, whereas Catherine describes the occupational therapist's role in trying to change attitudes in the community to develop social inclusion and to challenge discriminatory practice.

Part four, 'Special Issues Arising', is not about features necessarily unique to forensic services but issues exacerbated, or requiring greater attention than in general psychiatry, because of the nature of the work. Many occupational therapists know from bitter experience how difficult it can be to establish a service. Often occupational therapy is just an afterthought or so vaguely understood by others that it is a major struggle to fit comfortably into a positive working alliance with the full team. Gill Urquhart describes a positive experience of 'Setting up a forensic occupational therapy service' and how it was achieved. Security echoes through every chapter. Because it is perhaps the one issue which so demonstrably separates forensic from general mental health services, we felt it needed a chapter on its own. In 'Security issues for occupational therapists working in a medium secure setting' Andrea Neeson and Rebecca Kelly have written a useful guide for therapists new to the area. It may also be helpful to managers who need to consider the security implications of undertaking activities with mentally disordered offenders. 'Team working and liaison' are keys to successful forensic occupational therapy; Helena Holford and Deborah Alred discuss positive approaches to enhance good interdisciplinary practice.

Part five, 'Clinical Issues', considers occupational therapy with some specific groups of people. 'Women in secure environments' cannot properly be regarded as a clinical entity, but their care has been overlooked or crudely annexed to a male-orientated service. Kathryn Harris explains the background and suggests intervention strategies to enable gender-sensitive provision. Rachel Prentice and Kirsty Wilson recount why people with learning disabilities are, and should be, treated in separate specialist services. In their chapter 'Forensic occupational therapy within learning disability services', they indicate how the key principles of rights, independence, choice and inclusion are integrated in good practice. There are still significant numbers of people, mainly women, who remain detained in high secure settings despite having no forensic history. The behaviour that leads to their continued detention is nearly always that of self-injury. Ann McQue tackles this difficult topic in her chapter 'Self-injury or relief from overwhelming emotions'. 'Forensic addictive behaviours' too, we felt, merits its own chapter and so John Chacksfield has highlighted how the use of alcohol and drugs, or other addictive behaviours, adds another layer of complexity to the rehabilitation process. In 'Occupational therapy and the sexual offender' Edward Duncan acknowledges that few crimes elicit a stronger reaction from society than sexual offences do. Beyond the emotional response, he provides a detailed account of the occupational therapist's role with this client group and considers its potential development. Part five concludes with 'Personality disorder – a possible role for occupational therapy'. Lorna Couldrick indicates why people deemed psychopathic become like a hot potato, every service wishing to pass them on as quickly as possible, with a mixture of notions of how best to deal with them, from punishment, treatment to protection of society.

Recurring themes

Various issues reverberate throughout this book. The first of these is the nature of the client group. It consists of men and women whose ages range from 17 years to old age, although proportionately young men predominate. Some are admitted for 28 days only, for assessment, where as others will have been incarcerated in secure environments for decades. Some will be moving through the system to increasing levels of security yet the majority will eventually return, through decreasing levels of security, to the community. However, a minority will remain in prison or hospital for the rest of their lives. They demonstrate a wide range of mental disorders and some will be acutely ill, whilst others will not experience any symptoms of mental illness. They come from all walks of life but one thing remains almost universal: their lack of motivation and their difficult-to-engage nature. Forensic occupational therapy occurs at the interface of the criminal justice system and mental health legislation. The forensic client is held against his or her will or may be subject to restrictions in the community. Many have had no indication of how long this will be for. Lay people may see a mental health disposal for an offender as a soft option yet for the offender a pre-determined sentence of time can be infinitely easier to manage than to be held at Her Majesty's pleasure.

Another recurring theme is the tension between therapy versus containment. By the very nature of the work, risk assessment and security must be considered. Therapeutic work cannot occur in an unsafe environment, but rigid security measures can limit therapeutic intervention. Some have argued that security in some settings has gone too far (Chacksfield 2000). However, authors in this book share their clinical reasoning, demonstrating how they have struggled to address this tension. They also describe the value of working within a multiprofessional team, both for support and the sharing of expertise about this challenging client group. Working within a mutually supportive team appears to be one of the key factors in ensuring safety. This demands excellent communication between professions, confidence and trust to share skills, and respect for unique and specialist skills.

Likewise, reflection on practice and the need for a heightened self-awareness for the therapist also echoes throughout the book. To this end, several authors emphasize the importance of good-quality supervision and support. Particularly where therapists work in professional isolation, they do need to develop strong support systems. This may be across services, but can also be via the developing forensic networks.

Forensic occupational therapy networks

Forensic occupational therapy is a rapidly growing sphere of professional practice in the United Kingdom. This development, in such a specialized area, has given rise to supportive networks of occupational therapists throughout Great Britain. These include:

- the National and Regional Forensic Head Occupational Therapists Forums
- the Regional Research and Development Groups, organized by and for all grades of occupational therapy staff
- peer supervision and support across forensic units. These have resulted in shared initiatives and multicentre working
- the National Forensic Occupational Therapy Conference. This has been running successfully every year since 1998 and is organized by The State Hospital, Carstairs.

These groups are active in developing good practice within the speciality. For example, *The Standards for Practice for Occupational Therapy in Forensic Residential Settings* (College of Occupational Therapists 2002a) were compiled in collaboration with the National Forensic Head Occupational Therapy Forum and drew on the hard work of all staff who participated in the pilot study. These networks have also supported the development of this book.

We also live in an age where huge resources are available and opportunities exist for networking online. As a starting place, readers are recommended to visit the Forensic Nursing Resources Home Page (www.fnrh.freeserve.co.uk). This makes available many relevant documents and provides hyperlinks to other forensic sites, including journals, research collaborations and so on. There is also an emerging forensic occupational therapy internet discussion group. It is a forum for forensic occupational therapists to share ideas, ask questions and discuss professional issues. The web site, and joining instructions, can be found at *http://uk.groups.yahoo.com/group/forensic_occupational_therapy*

Satisfactions of working in forensic

Increasingly, in acute hospital services, the time available for rehabilitation is getting less and less. Therapists complain of the revolving door, with barely sufficient time to learn the patients' names before priority must be given to establishing they are safe for discharge. Even in community mental health teams, resource management means it can be difficult to justify long-term interventions. In forensic services, however, the one thing usually available is time. Time to undertake well-planned, in-depth rehabilitation. To work with a patient, so ill on admission that they are unable to manage basic personal care, and gradually plan a programme that equips them with the skills to live independently within their own bedsit is rewarding indeed.

There is also the joy of working as part of a dynamic and stimulating team. This is not just working alongside other professionals sharing a commitment to the health and welfare of the client. It is also to have other disciplines actively engaged in the activity programme, seeing its significance and wanting to be a part of it. A treasured memory is the transformation that occurred for one patient when she worked alongside her doctor in preparing a group meal. The registrar enjoyed bringing her family's favourite recipe for chicken curry to the group. The group, and in particular one female patient, valued the humility and humanity of the act of participation by a person previously held in awe and fear.

Moving on

Undeniably, much has been left out. For example, too late to rectify, we noticed we had included little on work or vocational rehabilitation and nothing on the varied cultural needs of the clients. We see this book as a beginning that we hope will be followed by many more books, where the ideas presented here can be refined and developed. Incorporated into these new texts will be the changes that we can foresee but which are not part of current practice. This includes the continuing implementation of the NHS Plan and the clinical governance agenda (Department of Health 1998, Department of Health 2000) and recently published professional standards of practice (College of Occupational Therapists 2002a). Additionally, new mental health legislation for Scotland, and England and Wales, is entering the statute book.

A review of the knowledge and research base for occupational therapy in forensic settings suggests 'that the canvas is almost blank, providing huge scope for a future agenda of research and development' (Mountain 1998 p.15). We intend this book to be a starting point, providing a baseline description of current practice. We hope it will encourage some to develop and challenge the themes emerging and inspire others to begin testing scientifically the observations described here. The National Programme on Forensic Mental Health Research and Development was established in April 1999 (Department of Health 2002). Copies of expert papers commissioned by the group are available on the Department of Health's website (www.doh.gov.uk/fmhrd). Likewise, the College of Occupational Therapists (2002b) has published its *Research and Development Strategic Vision and Action Plan for Forensic Occupational Therapy*. This identifies objectives for occupational and multidisciplinary enquiry and sets out a 10-year strategic framework. Additionally, the first research priorities exercise for forensic occupational therapy has now been completed. This outlines the research priority framework for this challenging area, as determined by practising clinicians (Duncan et al. 2003).

> Research is tremendously important, but it is a horse to be ridden and not a deity to be worshipped. At its best it can propel us into a more effective and assured future but, at its worst, it erodes the courage to say what we think without feeling obliged to prove that at least three other people have already said it.   (Willson 2002 p.312)

At present, there is little empirical evidence to support forensic occupational therapy practice, but that does not mean there is no evidence of efficacy. This book provides evidence gained through the experience of skilled practitioners.

Conclusion

We do hope you enjoy this book and that the experiences of forensic occupational therapists presented here will inform and stimulate discussion. Working in forensic services can be immensely rewarding. It can also be challenging and demanding. We see this book as a starting point and trust that it will be followed by many more. We are confident that future research will provide greater evidence for the ideas presented here. Research is important to provide sound evidence for practice. This will take time to achieve, however. In the meantime, we believe the following chapters will assist readers to understand and have confidence in the work of forensic occupational therapy.

References

Chacksfield J (2000) Patients must get therapeutic space. Therapy Weekly, 20 July 2000.

College of Occupational Therapists (1998) Occupational Therapy Services – Securing the Future? Executive summary of a conference held 12 March 1998. London: College of Occupational Therapists.

College of Occupational Therapists (2002a) The Standards for Practice: Occupational Therapy in Forensic Residential Settings. London: College of Occupational Therapists.

College of Occupational Therapists (2002b) Research and Development Strategic Vision and Action Plan for Forensic Occupational Therapy. London: College of Occupational Therapists.

Crawford M (1998) Current Occupational Therapy Activity and Staff Profiles in Forensic Psychiatry. Presented at Occupational Therapy Services – Securing the Future? Conference held 12 March 1998. London: College of Occupational Therapists.

Department of Health (1998) A First-class Service: Quality in the New NHS. London: The Stationery Office.

Department of Health (2000) The NHS Plan: A Plan for Investment, a Plan for Reform. London: The Stationery Office.

Department of Health (2002) National Programme on Forensic Mental Health Research and Development. Downloaded from http://www.doh.gov.uk/fmhrd.htm on 06/09/02.

Duncan E, Munro K and Nicol M (2003) Research priorities in forensic occupational therapy. The British Journal of Occupational Therapy 66(2) 55–64.

Lloyd C (1995) Forensic Psychiatry for Health Professionals. London: Chapman and Hall.

Mercer D, Mason T, McKeown M and McGann G (eds.) (2000) Forensic Mental Health Care: A Case Study Approach. Edinburgh: Churchill Livingstone.

Mountain G (1998) Occupational Therapy in Forensic Settings: A preliminary review of the knowledge and research base. London: Research and Development Group, College of Occupational Therapists.

Robinson D and Kettles A (eds.) (2000) Forensic Nursing and Multidisciplinary Care of Mentally Disordered Offenders. London: Jessica Kingsley.

Stone J, Roberts M, O'Grady J and Taylor A with O'Shea K (2000) Faulk's Basic Forensic Psychiatry (3rd edition). Oxford: Blackwell Science.

Willson M (2002) The Casson Memorial Lecture 2002: A Culture to Care For. British Journal of Occupational Therapy 65(7) 306–314.

Vaughan P and Badger D (1995) Working with the Mentally Disordered Offender in the Community. London: Chapman and Hall.

Webb D and Harris R (eds.) (1999) Mentally Disordered Offenders: Managing People Nobody Owns. London: Routledge.

CHAPTER 2

So what is forensic occupational therapy?

LORNA COULDRICK

Introduction

The number of occupational therapists working within forensic services in the United Kingdom has rapidly increased in the past two decades. This follows the *Butler Report* (Home Office and Department of Health and Social Security 1974), which recommended provision of medium secure beds in every region to provide staged levels of security and rehabilitation. These were the Regional Secure Units (RSU). The increase also reflects changing patterns of mental health service delivery following the development of community care and the closure of the asylums (Prior 1993). The consequent loss of locked wards combined with the public perception of increased risk of harm gave political impetus to provide improved services for the mentally disordered offender. Later the *Reed Report* (Department of Health and Home Office 1992) recommended an increase in medium secure provision, diversion of the mentally ill from the criminal justice system and improvements to the care of mentally disordered offenders, including rehabilitation. Alongside this expansion is the emerging perception of occupational therapy as a profession that can address some of the complex needs of mentally disordered offenders. The link between an individual's occupational performance, mental health and offending behaviour is increasingly being recognized.

One aim of this chapter is to clarify the different philosophy and value base of occupational therapy and why being busy is not, of its own, therapeutic. Another is to provide a rationale for the integration of these concepts into both interdisciplinary care plans for individual patients as well as organizational and strategic planning in forensic services. Occupational therapy is not offered as a 'cure all' approach and must be seen within the context of its unique contribution to the shared therapeutic endeavour of the interdisciplinary team. Similarly, not all activity will be undertaken by the occupational therapist; many others are also involved. This chapter distinguishes what makes activity therapeutic.

The chapter begins by exploring a definition of forensic occupational therapy and then separates the concept of being busy from the purposeful intention of occupational therapy. It argues that occupational therapists need to articulate better what it is they do. For too long the profession has been dogged by misunderstanding and confusion about its core purpose. To redress this, the underpinning beliefs and values of the profession are considered alongside some of the core skills.

Defining forensic occupational therapy

Defining *forensic* is relatively easy. In the *Concise Oxford Dictionary* it is defined as 'of or used in connection with courts of law'. Thus, forensic science describes that branch of science which is focused particularly on establishing evidence to be presented in court. Forensic psychiatry deals with the assessment, treatment, containment and community management of mentally disordered offenders.

Defining *occupational therapy* is less easy. The Canadian Association of Occupational Therapists consider that 'the primary role of occupational therapy is that of enabling occupation' (Townsend et al. 1997 p.30).

'Occupation is everything people do to occupy themselves, including looking after themselves (self-care), enjoying life (leisure), and contributing to the social and economic fabric of their communities (productivity)' (Townsend et al. 1997 p.30). When an individual is incarcerated, they are deprived of their former occupations. In reality, the very intent of forensic services is to prevent individuals engaging in some activities. However, the subsequent restrictions, and lack of choice of meaningful activity, results in occupational deprivation, which may lead to depression and apathy. Several chapters pick up this important theme, but avoiding occupational deprivation is only part of the forensic occupational therapist's role. There is another crucial element, that of harnessing the therapeutic effectiveness of engaging in occupations.

The College of Occupational Therapists provides the following definition:

'Occupational therapy is the treatment of people with physical and psychiatric illness or disability through specific selected occupation for the purpose of enabling individuals to reach their maximum level of function and independence in all aspects of life. The occupational therapist assesses the physical, psychological and social functions of the individual, identifies areas of dysfunction and involves the individual in a structured programme of activity to overcome disability. The activities selected will relate to the consumer's personal, social, cultural and economic needs and will reflect the environmental factors which govern his/her life' (College of Occupational Therapists 1994 p.2).

This book provides examples of how this definition translates into the practice of the forensic occupational therapist. This chapter considers the values and skill base that underpin their interventions. Of particular importance are two core beliefs of the profession: that occupation is fundamental and essential to human existence, and the value of occupation as a dynamic of therapy. These beliefs are developed further in differentiating being busy from the purposeful therapeutic intent of occupational therapy. It is argued that it is these two beliefs that distinguish the occupational therapy role from any other forensic health profession.

Although this book primarily addresses the professional contribution made in forensic psychiatry, assuming all forensic occupational therapy is directed toward the mentally disordered offender would be limiting. Certainly, at present, most occupational therapy in prison is with those who have mental health problems, but the links between occupational performance, alienation and offending behaviour are being recognized. A report by the Social Exclusion Unit (2002) suggests custodial sentences are not succeeding in turning the majority of prisoners away from crime. Many prisoners have very poor basic life skills and the report highlights that a prison sentence actually poses 'real dangers of mental and physical health deteriorating further, of life skills and thinking being eroded' (Social Exclusion Unit 2002 p.3). The report proposes that custodial sentences should be reformed to reduce reoffending. There is a role to be forged by forensic occupational therapists in helping to achieve this change.

Thus, forensic occupational therapy can be seen not only as the treatment of people with mental health problems who offend but also as a means of addressing offending behaviour. It is about acknowledging the important link between occupational behaviour and well-being. Helping people to engage in occupations that give their lives meaning and value and connect them to the society and culture in which they live not only promotes health but may mitigate alienation and antisocial behaviour.

Separation of being busy from occupational therapy

Throughout forensic services, different staff groups are involved in the use of activities either incidentally or as a major part of their role. This includes prison officers, technical instructors, nurses, psychologists and educationalists. The Special Hospitals were founded on Protestant work ethic principles, and the new rehabilitation services are growing from the old occupations departments, which were originally vocationally, or diversionary, based (Muth and Williams 1995). It is important to acknowledge and recognize that these activities are an essential, valuable part of the therapeutic regime. There are considerable overlaps and complementary practice with forensic occupational therapy. While acknowledging the contribution of others, this chapter outlines the specific nature of forensic occupational therapy.

A subtitle considered for this book was 'Using Time Not Doing Time', a phrase plagiarised from a lecture given by the then Chief Inspector of Prisons, Judge Stephen Tumin in 1994. He spoke eloquently of the futility of prisoners sewing mailbags or breaking rocks. Judge Tumin outlined his vision of prisoners using their time to equip them for a future less dependent on offending. As he spoke, it seemed he was outlining the role of the forensic occupational therapist. There is an absolute difference between using activity as punishment, as a means of atonement or as a way of managing dangerous people safely, and that of using activity as a therapeutic medium. To clarify this difference, it is necessary to look at the philosophical standpoint of the profession.

Professional philosophy is a system of *beliefs* or *values*. Values can be defined as one's principles or standards, one's judgement of what is valuable and important in life. Values are not rigidly fixed but evolve, through reason and argument, and are affected by culture and need. Many have tried to articulate the philosophy underpinning occupational therapy (Yerxa 1983, Mayers 1990, Kielhofner 1997, Townsend 1997, Wilcock 1998, Hagedorn 2001). Summarizing their work it may be said that occupational therapy believes in, or values:

- occupation as fundamental and essential to human existence
- occupation as a dynamic of therapy
- the humanity of the individual
- the individual's subjective experience.

These values are set in the conviction that the individual must be understood in the widest context of environment, family and culture.

Occupation is seen as fundamental and essential to human existence; that is, human beings have an occupational nature. Occupation is such a natural human phenomenon it is usually taken for granted because it forms the fabric of everyday lives. Throughout the ages, people have cited its value to health (Wilcock 2001). This is not exclusive to occupational therapy. The pioneers of the profession include doctors, nurses, social workers, master craftsmen, teachers and others who recognized the influence of occupation. Thus, it may be assumed, other professions do value occupation to varying degrees, but it seems that no other profession cites it as a core value. Activity is so fundamental, so obvious, it is seen in the background of the picture not as the object of the picture. Not so for occupational therapists; for them this value orders their professional learning and the priority of their work.

Detained patients and prisoners are inherently active within the limits of their environment, and many staff, intuitively, will engage in therapeutic activity. For example the key nurse who uses her gardening skills to build her relationship with a mistrustful and difficult-to-engage-with remand prisoner. Potting up the hanging baskets provides a safe non-threatening context in which to learn about each other. Other professions may facilitate activity but, for many, it has to come after their other duties of medication, security, etc. For occupational therapists, it is their priority. In the community, this may mean enabling the client to achieve a better balance of occupation through using local resources. In the secure environment, it is about changing the prisoner's or patient's experience from doing time to using time. This may be through learning social and life skills, for example, or using creative activity as an acceptable way of expressing distressing thoughts and feelings.

The second value – of occupation and activity as a dynamic of therapy – frames the knowledge and skills base of the profession. This has grown from the expertise acquired in the application of occupation. However, this tacit 'knowing in action' (Schon 1991) is not easily articulated. Sometimes, the activity is erroneously measured by the product or artefact rather than by the process. It is frustrating to hear the wobbly, asymmetrical pot criticized, or praise heaped upon a workshop that delivers superb professionally crafted wooden toys, when there has been no analysis of whether the work engendered was therapeutic. It is the process of undertaking the activity, the therapeutic dynamic, which the profession has, since its inception, tried to define and validate.

Experience suggests that others often neither understand the dynamic nor appreciate the core skills required to ensure therapeutic success. An example is a group activity with mentally disordered offenders; the task, to cook a meal for the community within the secure environment. Another member of staff is keen to be involved and efficiently, but in isolation, prepares the vegetables. Careful explanation is needed that the goal is not the production of the meal in the most efficient manner. The purpose is the relationship fostered between patients and staff as they work with a common purpose together. This includes: the return to the patient of some element of control, the provision of a sense of involvement and belonging to the community, the provision of social opportunity whereby the patient must practise skills of negotiation and cooperation within the group and the sense of achievement and self-esteem at the successful completion of the task.

Being engaged in activity, being busy, is not in itself therapeutic. In many forensic settings, the covert purpose of activity may be the safe management of behaviour. Where activity occurs off the ward, patients may be encouraged to participate without any clear sense of purpose other than providing relief for the ward-based staff (Muth and Williams 1995). More often, it is the lack of thought or analysis of activity that can make it damaging rather than helpful.

Computer games, for example, can be an ideal way to engage a disturbed patient. On first admission to a secure setting some offenders pace in wide circuits around the room, watching but unwilling, or unable, to speak or relate to any other person in the room. The computer game may provide a quick attention-grabbing medium. Well used, this can be subtly employed to develop trust and rapport. The game must be appropriate for the individual and at a level for quick success. Sadly, examples abound of computer games being badly used. Perhaps a too complicated or demanding game was chosen or the staff member begins to compete against the patient, further damaging their fragile sense of self. Or worse still, the staff member becomes absorbed in the game ignoring the patient. Certainly, this last approach led one patient to smash the computer!

A belief in the humanity of the individual is not unique to occupational therapy. It is, however, an important value in the forensic setting and can be extremely difficult to achieve. It has been described as the deeply ingrained sense of each person's worth, irrespective of any impairment (Kielhofner 1997). It is allied to client-centred notions of non-judgemental positive regard (Rogers 1967). It is a challenging concept because, by the very nature of forensic work, the client group has offended society, breached its rules of right and decency. The value demands that the therapist must endeavour to see beyond the offence to the individual and engage with him or her to understand better their offending, and often offensive, behaviour.

Likewise, some other professions share valuing the individual's subjective experience. It is about trying to empathize with, and understand, the individual's lived experience, hearing his or her narrative. Endeavouring to access their inner world can be difficult. Sometimes it is also a painful and disturbing process for the therapist, but it is essential for building a working alliance, without which occupational therapy cannot occur. Occupational therapy, unlike some other interventions such as medication, cannot be administered without cooperation from the patient. Valuing the individual's subjective experience is not condoning or making allowance for behaviour but trying to hear the offender's perspective.

The need to articulate better the intention of occupational therapy

It can be difficult for others to see the uniqueness of occupational therapy, and three inherent reasons are suggested that can contribute to this lack of understanding. First, it is because the link between human occupation, health and well-being is so fundamental that it is barely talked about, let alone carefully analysed, assessed and recorded. It is little wonder that the interdisciplinary team may not appreciate the therapeutic intent of the activity chosen. Or the patient's engagement in occupation is diminished to two words at his or her review: 'milieu therapy'. We urge occupational therapists to publicize their work to other professional groups. In order for patient care teams to understand the therapeutic nature of the endeavour it must be clearly linked to the patient's identified needs and the clinical benefits explicitly stated.

Second, the activity is so ordinary and everyday. Other professions have major, obvious and specialist tasks unique to their role, for example prescribing or administering medication, ensuring security, legal management, etc. Or they undertake tasks seen as requiring particular proficiency such as the authorization to administer a personality inventory or the mysteries of psychotherapy. On the other hand, occupational therapists do mundane, ordinary activities. Creek (1996) exemplifies this in her article 'Making a Cup of Tea as an Honours Degree Subject'. She compares the apparent simplicity of the task of making a cup of tea with the richness, sophistication and versatility of this activity. To the lay observer any person could undertake these mundane, simple activities. For the occupational therapist it may demand subtle skills to motivate, the ability to analyse the complexity of the activity, an aptitude to adapt the activity to address identified needs, an understanding of the actual and symbolic meanings of that activity to the client, plus expertise to address balance in occupation.

Third, an enabling role should minimize the achievement of the therapist and maximize the achievement of the patient. The better occupational therapists are at their job, the less their contribution should be seen. That is, if the occupational therapist works well, his or her part in the activity should be imperceptible while the client's achievement should be evident. Success is the patient having a sense of mastery, not the feeling that their therapist has worked particularly hard to make this happen. To illustrate, during my time at Ashen Hill a charge nurse once commented that when I undertook the group meal it always achieved high levels of patient participation. He attributed this to my personality. What I had failed to explain was my complex clinical reasoning in planning the task. From the moment of the proposal to cook a meal for the unit to its execution, I would be thinking and planning the activity. I would match skill levels to task. A more disturbed patent might be invited to come into the kitchen and work, one to one, at a discrete achievable task prior to the main group event. Some patients would need subtle, gentle encouragement, whereas others were able to lead the group. In this event, they would be cast as head chef, with me as their lackey.

The skills of the forensic occupational therapist

Many texts outline the skills of the occupational therapist (College of Occupational Therapists 1994, Finlay 1997, Creek 1997, Hagedorn 2001) so attention here will be given only to four skills, as they relate to forensic occupational therapy. These include:

- the skills to motivate
- task analysis, grading and application
- understanding the meaning of the activity to the client
- occupational balance.

Every forensic occupational therapist must, at the core of their practice, have advanced *motivational skills*. Forensic clients are compulsorily detained in secure environments or, in the community, are subject to restriction orders and enforced monitoring. They often have angry hostile relationships with people in authority including health professionals. This can be expressed overtly in aggressive behaviour or covertly in passive resistance. Therefore, they can be notoriously difficult to engage and by choice they may prefer to remain isolated and in bed. Motivation on a unit can spiral downwards. The therapist invests time and effort in planning a new group; a proportion of patients lacks the motivation to attend; the therapist takes less effort with the next group; it is less interesting for the participants, fewer attend. I suspect most seasoned forensic occupational therapists have experienced times when the whole activity programme has collapsed.

Not only must the occupational therapist be able to motivate the client, he or she must also be able to re-motivate themselves. A patient's behaviour may evoke hostile feelings in staff causing them to lose motivation. Additionally, the occupational therapist may need to motivate and energize other members of the staff group as the full richness of the programme depends on the participation of many. All staff engaged in activity need support, supervision and encouragement.

Task analysis, grading and application can be illustrated by drawing on an experience of a negative example of anti-therapeutic activity. A small group of well-intentioned staff tried to engage a client in a workshop activity beyond his present ability. The task, building a doll's house, was complex and lengthy. The patient was surfacing from a period of debilitating depression. Each day he was escorted to the workshop where well-meaning assistance was given. The effect, however, was that the patient observed staff doing what he felt he was unable to do. His feelings of uselessness were reinforced. The timescale to completion meant that this experience was repeated daily for several weeks. It became a test of endurance. People with depression need immediate success. The task must offer some intrinsic positive feedback at least within 20 minutes. Many small successes can build to a therapeutic larger activity, but this requires skills to break down the task into sequenced, manageable components.

When activities are carefully analysed, they can be used in versatile and creative ways to meet the various assessed needs of the client. For example, art can be used to develop leisure skills. Alternatively, it may provide a vehicle to practise social skills. Or it may be used projectively to explore the client's inner world. Likewise, cooking may be just ten minutes' popping corn to provide instant positive success as a first step in building self-esteem. Or it may be carefully graded and structured to prepare someone to return to his or her own home in the community. Or, as seen earlier, it can be used for the group meal where there is no intention of developing culinary expertise. These differences need to be clearly specified and understood by the patient care team.

A mantra of the occupational therapist is that *activity must be meaningful* to the client. Thus, the occupational therapist requires an ingrained sense of the symbolic and actual meanings of the activity for the client. Is gardening a chore, a monotonous drudge or an activity that inspires a spiritual sense of the cyclical nature of life and regrowth? The activity must relate to the client's cultural values and belief.

Occupational balance is raised in several chapters. All occupational therapists are concerned about the balance between the three elements of productivity, self-care and leisure. For the forensic occupational therapist, balance has an additional element: therapeutic balance. Unlike most other settings, the patient's time is managed 24 hours a day, and thought needs to be given to the totality of each person's programme. Various activities and media may promote different skills and challenges. Working towards achieving NVQ level 3 in a trade may be infinitely valuable to the patient's future employment prospects but this is nothing if no attention has been paid to offending behaviour. Likewise, some patients may be participating in intense psychotherapy or undertaking activities that encourage introspection and painful journeys of self-discovery. They too need the balance of activities that allows them relief from morbid preoccupation. Frequently, balance must include physical activity to overcome the inertia and lethargy of a secure environment.

Before closing on skills, it is worth considering interprofessional working. Each team member has profession-specific skills plus skills shared by other professions. Some individuals then add to these advanced specialist skills. Thus many of the team may have excellent motivational skills, but that does not mean, for example, all nurses, doctors or psychologists must be good motivators. However, I would consider it an essential core skill for every forensic occupational therapist. Similarly, all therapeutic activity is not undertaken solely by the occupational therapist. Indeed, drawing on the interests and resources of the team can enrich the whole activity programme. However, occupational therapy is the only profession that puts it at the core of its purpose.

Conclusion

No one is inactive. All human beings engage in activity, including those detained in a secure environment. However, activity in itself is not necessarily therapeutic, it may even be harmful. A patient may withdraw and isolate themselves in their activity, they may become excessively busy to avoid looking at painful inner conflicts or they may be encouraged to undertake a task beyond their ability, thus reinforcing their negative self-concept. Understanding the nature of activity – how it relates to personal value systems, skills of task analysis and the ability to motivate, engage and implement activity at appropriate levels to the client – are core skills of occupational therapy. Additionally, forensic occupational therapists are helping people engage in occupations that give their lives meaning and value and connect them to the society and culture in which they live. This not only promotes health but may mitigate alienation and antisocial behaviour.

References

College of Occupational Therapists (1994) Core Skills and a Conceptual Framework for Practice: A Position Statement. London: College of Occupational Therapists.

Creek J (ed.) (1997) Occupational Therapy and Mental Health (2nd edition). Edinburgh: Churchill Livingstone.

Creek J (1996) Making a cup of tea as an honours degree subject. British Journal of Occupational Therapy 59(3) 128–130.

Department of Health and Home Office (1992) Review of Health and Social Services for Mentally Disordered Offenders and Others Requiring Similar Services, chaired by Dr John Reed. Final Summary Report. London: HMSO.

Finlay L (1997) The Practice of Psychosocial Occupational Therapy (2nd edition). Cheltenham: Stanley Thornes.

Hagedorn R (2001) Foundations for Practice in Occupational Therapy (3rd edition). Edinburgh: Churchill Livingstone.

Home Office and Department of Health and Social Security (1974) Interim Report of the Committee on Mentally Abnormal Offenders. (The Butler Committee). London: HMSO.

Kielhofner G (1997) The Conceptual Foundations of Occupational Therapy (2nd edition). Philadelphia: F. A. Davis Company.

Mayers C (1990) A philosophy unique to occupational therapy. British Journal of Occupational Therapy 53(9) 379–380.

Muth Z and Williams R (Eds) (1995) With Care in Mind Secure: A review for the Special Hospitals Service Authority of the services provided by Ashworth Hospital. Sutton: Health Advisory Service.

Prior L (1993) The Social Organisation of Mental Illness. London: Sage Publications.

Rogers C (1967) On Becoming a Person: A Therapist's View of Psychotherapy. London: Constable.

Schon D (1991) The Reflective Practitioner: How Professionals Think in Action. Aldershot: Arena.

Social Exclusion Unit (2002) Reducing Re-Offending by Ex-Prisoners. London: Social Exclusion Unit.

Townsend E (ed.) (1997) Enabling Occupation: An Occupational Therapy Perspective. Ottawa: CAOT Publications.

Wilcock A (1998) An Occupational Perspective of Health. Thorofare NJ: Slack Inc.

Wilcock A (2001) Occupation for Health, Volume I. London: British Association and College of Occupational Therapists.

Yerxa E (1983) Audacious values: The energy source for occupational therapy Practice. In: Health Through Occupation: Theory and Practice in Occupational Therapy, Kielhofner G (ed.). Philadelphia: F. A. Davis and Co.

CHAPTER 3
The foundation of good practice

MARION MARTIN

Why use theory?

Many students and practitioners of occupational therapy question the value of theory. It could be argued that effective interventions can be carried out without wasting time on trying to understand and apply frames of reference and models of practice to our work. However, the increasing demand for professionals to explain and justify what they do is encouraging practitioners to reflect on the underlying rationale for their work in any particular setting.

Theories are often criticized for being too complex and laden with jargon and that they serve only to make a relatively straightforward intervention unnecessarily complicated. However, it is vital that forensic occupational therapists get to grips with important ideas that have a powerful influence over what they do. This is because, by the very nature of working in a secure environment, the forensic occupational therapist is within a closed institution working with people who have extremely complex needs. Institutions acquire an ethos, an approach, and it is essential that occupational therapists understand not only what beliefs underpin this approach but also how it fits with their preferred way of working.

A good example of the relevance of theory to our work, especially in forensic settings, is the nature–nurture controversy. The nature side of the argument holds that people are genetically predisposed to behave in the way that they do, so that in the case of a criminal the implications are that only radical measures such as the death penalty, lifetime incarceration, medication or surgery would be indicated. The theory of nurture, on the other hand, acknowledges the influence that the environment has on the individual, with the implication that rehabilitation is possible through a more supportive environment. These two positions are not nearly as simple as I have presented them here, but may begin to explain why there are different attitudes towards the treatment of those who have committed a serious crime and those who are mentally ill (Prins 1995, Pilgrim and Rogers 1999).

Occupational therapists can also use theory to help to explain to others what they are doing and why they are doing it. By its nature, occupational therapy can often look simplistic and may for this reason be undervalued. For example, a game of football or a cooking group is more likely to be interrupted by other staff than a meeting with the social worker. This is because it is the activity alone that is seen and not what the activity is being used to achieve. An understanding of the theory underpinning practice can assist forensic occupational therapists in justifying what makes their approach unique.

Finlay (1997) identifies four ways in which theory can be used: as a guide to practice, as a guide to alternative practice, as a tool to encourage team cooperation, and as a way forward for the profession. She then warns the reader that 'there is much confusion and corresponding debate surrounding definitions of terms such as models, theories, approaches, frames of reference' (Finlay 1997 p.16). My own advice to the reader would be not to become too concerned with the type of theory but to try to understand some of the ideas and how they relate to your own experiences.

Historical perspective

When looking at occupational therapy theory, it helps to begin with a historical perspective. The founders of the profession described the objectives of the American National Society for the Promotion of Occupational Therapy in 1917 as, 'the advancement of occupation as a therapeutic measure; the study of the effect of occupation upon the human being; and the scientific dispensation of this knowledge' (cited in Wilcock 1998 p.167).

Since that time there has been very little 'study of the effect of occupation on the human being' or 'scientific dispensation of this knowledge'.

For some time, occupational therapy stopped promoting its fundamental beliefs, probably because they were not based on any research: it had not been carried out. The profession adopted the underlying rationale of other disciplines, especially medicine because it was more scientific. Occupational therapists increasingly found it difficult to describe their profession to others and articulate what exactly was their unique role (Yerxa 2000). In the physical field, the patient became a passive recipient of reductionistic intervention in order to facilitate rapid discharge from hospital. In mental health, occupational therapists preferred talking therapies such as counselling and cognitive behavioural therapy, using assistants to run the activities.

It was during the 1980s that occupational therapy became interested in models of practice in order to analyse and justify their work. By this time, they felt it was necessary to develop their own models rather than borrowing them from other professions such as medicine. Models bring together many fundamental concepts, such as holistic, client-centred practice, and combine them to make a coherent framework within which therapists can design assessments and plan their intervention.

The occupational therapy models of practice most widely applied are the Adaptation through Occupation Model (Reed and Sanderson 1999), the Canadian Model of Occupational Performance (Canadian Association of Occupational Therapists 1991, Townsend 1997) and the Model of Human Occupation (Kielhofner 1995). Succinct summaries of these can be found in books by Rosemary Hagedorn (2001) and Linda Finlay (1997) who use mental health case studies to deepen understanding. These models share certain core values of occupational therapy, namely, placing the individual at the centre of interacting systems so that any therapy has to be client centred, and emphasizing the importance of occupation to enable the client to adapt to their environment. Practitioners have found generic models such as these more useful to the occupational therapist working in a forensic setting than more specific approaches, as the needs of this client group are so diverse. Together with their associated assessments, such models can be used to structure a plan of intervention and analyse outcomes. The potential for using the Model of Human Occupation is discussed by Eddie Duncan in the chapter on occupational therapy and the sexual offender. Lorna Couldrick describes the use of the Adaptations through Occupations Model, in the chapter 'Personality disorder – a possible role for occupational therapy'.

Frames of reference and their associated approaches are used within models of practice according to the needs of the individuals concerned and the context within which intervention occurs. The approaches used most commonly in mental health are the psychodynamic, the humanistic, the behavioural, the cognitive behavioural, and with people with personality disorders, therapeutic communities. Rebecca Kelly, in her chapter, describes how she uses cognitive behavioural therapy within group work. Again, the reader is directed towards authors such as Hagedorn (2001) and Finlay (1997) for summaries of these theories, and to Cullen and Jones (1997) for therapeutic communities. It is important to understand the underlying assumptions of the different approaches, since in many ways they conflict with each other. Where members of the team are using contrasting methods of intervention, it is likely to lead to poor outcomes. These can include the non-integration of occupational therapy into the team as well as confusion and distress for the client.

Within the wider forensic team the approaches, frames of reference or models chosen determine the type of intervention used. It is possible to imagine a scenario where the nurses are using a behavioural programme and so are ignoring 'inappropriate' behaviour, the psychotherapist is using analytical group work and is encouraging the expression of anger, the doctors are using medication to subdue the active symptoms, and the occupational therapist is using a humanistic approach, encouraging clients to express themselves through their paintings. Each professional will have different expectations of the clients, who will be confused as to whether they have to be quiet and well behaved or to freely express their emotions. The experience of forensic occupational therapists suggests that a good understanding of the underlying assumptions of each profession is essential. Where this mutual understanding is achieved, teams can work cooperatively, and interventions complement each other. Where the ethos remains unsynchronized, teamwork can be poor, disjointed and hard to achieve.

Occupational science

By the 1990s, the relatively new profession of occupational therapy was coming of age. Certain therapists realized that the core beliefs of the founders offered an important and potentially revolutionary way of looking at health which had never been explored in any depth (Whiteford et al. 2000). This was the inception of occupational science. Readers wishing to find out more about this subject are recommended to seek out Zemke and Clark (1996), Clark et al. (1998) and the work of Ann Wilcock (1998, 2001 and 2002).

The occupational therapist in a forensic environment is in an excellent position to use occupations fully as therapy. Whereas occupational therapists in more acute settings find that they do not have the time to carry out an holistic assessment and plan of intervention, forensic occupational therapists are able to do this. In fact, when they are asked, it is this issue of having more time that is the most important reason cited for why practitioners choose to work in the secure services. There is time to develop a therapeutic relationship with the client and the opportunity to provide comprehensive occupational therapy programmes.

Whereas many occupational therapists may claim that the profession has had a lack of direction since its early days, writers on the role of occupational therapy in forensic settings have, over the years, adhered to a strong emphasis on important core values. Lloyd, in 1987, writes:

> The application of purposeful task engagement distinguishes occupational therapy from other mental health professionals working in the areas of forensic psychiatry. There is a need for occupational therapy to create a stimulating and challenging environmental setting for the patients they are treating in order to elicit exploratory behaviour thereby developing a sense of personal competence in the carrying out of personal life tasks and roles.
>
> (Lloyd 1987 p.24)

Writers on occupational science claim that humans have a need to be engaged in some form of occupation, not only to survive but also to thrive. When we feel anxious or threatened, we have an instinctive drive to be engaged in some form of activity, be it housework or computer games. Leisure activities, as well as work occupations, can bring about a feeling of well-being or 'flow'. Csikszentmihalyi (1992, 1997) describes flow as an 'optimal experience' which occurs when we are so involved in the activity that we lose ourselves in it. Those who frequently experience flow develop a stronger, more confident self. Flow occurs when both the challenges and skills are perceived by the individual to be at the highest levels, be it writing a poem or scoring a goal. The opposite of flow is apathy, boredom or anxiety. Under these circumstances, people are more likely to become unwell or to carry out socially unacceptable behaviour, as studies of unemployment have shown (Wilcock 1998).

Occupational therapists are in an ideal position, with their skills of activity analysis and clinical reasoning, to provide opportunities for flow to occur. The challenge, however, for those working in forensic units is that very often their clients have already experienced mastery and flow in anti-social activities before admission; they may have been the teenage gang-leader or the prison 'supremo', using their skills in physical violence or engendering fear in others. The occupational therapist's work is not just about keeping people busy. It involves a deep understanding of the client, including what motivates them, and how they perceive their own strengths, then combining this with a therapeutic programme which offers occupations that they will find demanding but are within their capabilities.

Occupational deprivation

Another challenge for the therapist working in a forensic setting is occupational deprivation, which is, 'a state of preclusion from engagement in occupations of necessity and/or meaning due to factors that stand outside the immediate control of the individual' (Whiteford 2000 p.201).

A central premise of occupational deprivation is that the circumstances that prevent someone from carrying out their chosen activities are beyond their control. This is, of course, the case for a client in a forensic setting for whom freedom of choice to be there has been denied, either for their own safety or that of the public.

Brenda Flood (1997) outlines the factors limiting practice within the forensic setting. She identifies: security and limited access to the community, reduced access to resourses, such as pieces of equipment or escorts, which can reduce participation in activities, and clients' low motivation, as they perceive that they have little control over their lives. The picture painted is that of occupational deprivation, as depicted by Whiteford

(1997, 2000). Consistent with other writers on the subject, Flood advocates the importance of choice of activity for the client in order to develop some feeling of control.

The number of occupational therapists working in secure units has increased rapidly in recent years, leading to a much richer experience for the client who is obliged to spend time in these establishments. One of the main concerns of these therapists now is for people once they are discharged into the community. On the unit, clients have a range of opportunities for meaningful activity, with supportive staff, but once they are granted their 'freedom' there is a possibility that they will return to an impoverished and hostile environment. This is the challenge described by Catherine Joe in her chapter on the development of community forensic occupational therapy.

Farnworth et al. (1987) and Whiteford (1997) have studied the work of occupational therapists in prison and also speak of the therapists' aim to improve their clients' self-esteem and help them to experience feelings of self-control. People with a history of continual failure are more likely to become demoralized and feel they have little control over the events in their lives. This may be one reason why they attempt deviant methods of attaining their goals. An essential principle of the occupational therapist's practice should be that the individual has the power, within limits agreed by the team, to determine their choice of activity, as well as the degree of difficulty posed (Farnworth et al. 1987).

The future

In addition to ameliorating the mental health of their clients, forensic occupational therapists have a responsibility towards society to address the antisocial behaviour that resulted in the client's admission to the service in the first place. The role of the occupational therapist in this setting is a complex one and will stretch them to the limits of their ability. For this reason, it can also be a very satisfying role. Occupational therapy theory is developing to assist professionals with their work, but a lot more evidence is required to help those who work in forensic units. More research is needed to establish the links between occupation and the origins of mental illness and crime. We need to understand the ways in which occupations can be used in the community as well as on forensic units to reduce mental illness and recidivism. In future occupational therapists could be used as consultants for crime prevention policy and contribute to the design of a healthier society.

Conclusion

Busy occupational therapists may not feel that they have enough time to digest the many different theoretical concepts that are being produced with ever-increasing abundance in recent years. However, it is recommended that they attempt to do so, as professionals are increasingly required to account for the decisions they make in their practice.

Occupational therapy originated from the belief that people can be healed through carrying out occupations that they find meaningful. This conviction was based more on intuition than on evidence. Although the founders of the profession articulated this principle very clearly, their successors found it more difficult to do so as they increasingly based their practice on the theoretical ideas of other professions such as medicine and psychology. In the 1980s, occupational therapists started developing models of practice that incorporated their core beliefs such as client-centred, holistic interventions. These models are particularly useful in forensic settings, as occupational therapists working in this environment are required to cover a vast range of issues concerning their clients.

Frames of reference can also help therapists in forensic settings to identify the approaches they are using in relation to the other members of their multiprofessional team. This may give them insight into possible team problems and help them to identify ways of working more effectively together. In recent years there has been a renewed interest in the role that occupation plays in people's lives, and a new discipline, occupational science, has emerged which encourages research into the healing properties of being active. Occupational therapists working in forensic settings have traditionally held values that are consistent with occupational science. They have been aware of the low self-esteem evident in their clients who have experienced little control over their lives, and of the importance of giving them choice over their occupational activity. They have acknowledged that these people are usually unmotivated to take part in any therapeutic programme, therefore any activities provided must be challenging and have meaning for them.

Occupational science teaches us that not only can occupational deprivation in prisons and other forensic environments lead to apathy, and ultimately to depression and ill health, but also it is likely that it may be one of the main causes of antisocial behaviour. It is our responsibility as occupational therapists to raise awareness of these issues at all levels, from the multiprofessional team to the makers of social policy, if we are to change the rising levels of crime in our society and to rehabilitate offenders, particularly those with identified mental health problems.

References

Canadian Association of Occupational Therapists (1991) Occupational Therapy Guidelines for Client-centred Practice. Toronto: Canadian Association of Occupational Therapists Publications.

Clark F, Wood W and Larson E (1998) Occupational science: Occupational therapy's legacy for the 21st century. In: Willard & Spackman's Occupational Therapy (9th edition), Neistadt M and Blesedell-Crepeau E (eds.). Philadelphia: J B Lippincott-Raven.

Csikszentmihalyi M (1992) Flow: The Psychology of Happiness. London: Rider.

Csikszentmihalyi M (1997) Living Well: The Psychology of Everyday Life. London: Harper Collins.

Cullen E and Jones L (1997) Therapeutic Communities for Offenders. Wiley series in Offender Rehabilitation. Chichester: John Wiley & Sons.

Farnworth L, Morgan S and Fernando B (1987) Prison-based occupational therapy. Australian Journal of Occupational Therapy 34(2) 40–46.

Finlay L (1997) The Practice of Psychosocial Occupational Therapy (2nd edition). Cheltenham: Stanley Thornes Publications.

Flood B (1997) An introduction to occupational therapy in forensic psychiatry. British Journal of Therapy and Rehabilitation 4(7) 375–380.

Hagedorn R (2001) Foundations for Practice in Occupational Therapy (3rd edition). Edinburgh: Churchill Livingstone.

Kielhofner G (ed.) (1995) Human Occupation: Theory and Application (2nd edition). Baltimore: Williams & Wilkins.

Lloyd C (1987) The role of occupational therapy in the treatment of the forensic psychiatric patient. Australian Occupational Therapy Journal 34(1) 20–25.

Pilgrim D and Rogers A (1999) A Sociology of Mental Health and Illness (2nd edition). Buckingham: Open University Press.

Prins H (1995) Offenders, Deviants or Patients? (2nd edition). London: Routledge.

Reed K and Sanderson S (1999) Concepts of Occupational Therapy (4th edition). Philadelphia: Lippincott, Williams & Wilkins.

Townsend E (ed.) (1997) Enabling Occupation: An Occupational Therapy Perspective. Ottawa: Canadian Association of Occupational Therapists.

Whiteford G (2000) Occupational deprivation: Global challenge in the new millennium. British Journal of Occupational Therapy 63(5) 200–204.

Whiteford G (1997) Occupational deprivation and incarceration. Journal of Occupational Science: Australia 6(3) 124–130.

Whiteford G, Townsend E and Hocking C (2000) Reflections on a renaissance of occupation. Canadian Journal of Occupational Therapy 67(1) 61–69.

Wilcock A (1998) An Occupational Perspective of Health. Thorofare NJ: Slack Inc.

Wilcock A (2001) Occupation for Health: Volume 1. London: British Association and College of Occupational Therapists.

Wilcock A (2002) Occupation for Health: Volume 2. London: British Association and College of Occupational Therapists.

Yerxa E (2000) Confessions of an occupational therapist who became a detective. British Journal of Occupational Therapy 63(5) 192–200.

Zemke R and Clark R (1996) Occupational Science: The Evolving Discipline. Philadelphia: FA Davis Co.

PART TWO

THE OCCUPATIONAL THERAPY PROCESS IN A MEDIUM SECURE UNIT

CHAPTER 4
Assessment

CLAIRE BARTON

Introduction

Assessment is an integral component of the occupational therapy process and allows the therapist to consider how the needs and abilities of the patient are influenced by the environment and the consequent impact upon the patient's quality of everyday life (Kielhofner 1997). Throughout a patient's admission the therapist is involved in assessment, utilizing the findings to grade intervention plans to ensure the patient's maintenance and, where possible, development of skills (Hagedorn 1995). While this remains consistent across all clinical fields, within the forensic setting the process becomes more complex due to the multifaceted needs of the patient group (Vaughan and Done 2000), the involvement of the Home Office and issues of security and risk.

This chapter provides detail of the assessment process and offers occupational therapists practical information regarding the selection and implementation of appropriate assessment tools for the forensic setting. For others, it helps to clarify the unique focus of the occupational therapist's assessment. It draws on personal experience to illustrate how theory may be usefully applied to practice. Relaying and recording the assessment, both to the patient and the clinical team, is also considered.

Assessment – a shared skill

Within the Bracton Centre, all members of the multidisciplinary team are involved in the assessment of patients. What is unique to occupational therapy, however, is first the use of activity as an assessment medium in itself. This requires sound observational skills and an astute ability to analyse activity. Second, the focus on functional skills must be considered, that is how individuals cope with work, leisure and self-care. Forensic occupational therapists need to be familiar with, and a appropriately from, the growing number of assessment tool: and reveal a patient's occupational performance.

Why assess?

Assessment, in itself, does not improve the patient's abilities but it does:

1. encourage the patient's active involvement in their care, promoting more favourable outcomes (Law et al. 1998) and is upheld by Standard 4 of the National Service Framework (Department of Health 1998)
2. enhance the therapist's understanding of the patient and the patient's understanding of themselves. This information, communicated to the multiprofessional team, also assists a more complete risk assessment (Snowden 1997, Fuller and Cowan 1999)
3. allow the therapist to establish a baseline of the patient's abilities and needs
4. assist the therapist and patient to set realistic goals enabling an individualized intervention plan to be drawn up
5. allow progress to be objectively monitored when utilizing sound assessment tools (McAdam et al. 2001); the need for evidence-based care makes it imperative that therapists can demonstrate effective interventions (Seally 1999)
6. help to define the parameters of the occupational therapist's role, input and skills to both the multiprofessional team and to the patient.

What to assess?

The College of Occupational Therapists (1995) offers guidelines for the assessment of patients with mental health needs. Areas for assessment include: self-care, work activities, leisure, social/interpersonal skills, cognitive skills and activities of daily living. All methods of assessment should be appropriate to the age, gender, cultural background and the patient's level of functioning (Standard 3). The future plans and goals of the patient, for example where the patient will be discharged to, need to be considered along with the skills necessary for the patient to function successfully in the community and have a reasonable quality of life. For instance, if a patient has never worked, does not wish to work and prefers to attend a day centre upon discharge, the assessment of employment skills is not appropriate. Within the forensic setting, the therapist will also be involved in the continuing process of risk assessment.

When to assess?

A prominent feature of operational policy within the forensic setting will be the maintenance of a secure environment and the assessment and management of risk. Both the Home Office and the clinical team will restrict the patient's activities until a greater understanding of the potential risks has been ascertained. Assessment opportunities, therefore, will depend upon the patient's progress and the risk management plan *in situ*.

Assessment is an ongoing feature of the occupational therapist's work, utilizing both formal and informal methods. In the early stages of a patient's admission, informal assessment may be most beneficial in allowing the therapist to establish a rapport with the patient, for example use of observational and listening skills while playing a game of pool. Such an approach can be less threatening and allows the development of a therapeutic relationship. More formal assessments, such as a structured interview, are better undertaken when a degree of trust has been established. It is not unusual for some patients to take several months to progress to the stage where formal assessment is possible.

During the initial stages of admission, the patient may be extremely unwell and experiencing florid first-rank psychotic symptoms including auditory or tactile hallucinations and delusions. The appropriateness of administering a formal assessment at this time is debatable. The patient is likely to demonstrate poor concentration, which can impair performance and may not accurately reflect the patient's abilities when well. The impact of underperforming can be particularly damaging to self-esteem and thus should be considered very carefully. On the other hand, informal assessment of the patient's abilities when unwell may enhance the risk management strategy, for example the patient who tends to neglect themselves when unwell may need increased domiciliary support.

Upon admission, the patient may commence a trial of medication, which can have unpleasant side effects including blurred vision, hypersalivation, drowsiness, lethargy, tremors and postural hypertension. These side effects can cause discomfort, embarrassment and may significantly impair performance in everyday activities. From experience, before assessing the patient, it is useful to check what medications are being administered and whether any side effects have been noted. The time the session occurs may be especially important if the side effects are more pronounced at particular times of the day, for example increased drowsiness in the morning.

Methods of assessment

Five basic assessment methods have been identified: structured observation, performance checks, interview, self-rating and standardized tests (Wilson 1987, Finlay 1997). The choice of assessment should complement the philosophy of the service and the occupational therapy model adopted. Some practice models, like the Model of Human Occupation (MoHO), have developed a comprehensive range of well-researched assessment tools as well as providing a theoretical framework to guide practice (Kielhofner 1997). Patients may find some approaches more helpful than others; for example, they may become increasingly anxious in formal situations such as sitting in an interview room but less so when walking in the garden. Hence, a flexible approach to assessment is beneficial. Culture, age and gender influence the patient's beliefs, values and practices. Therefore, awareness and understanding of these issues is essential to avoid misunderstandings and invalid assessment findings (Buchan 2002).

Assessment through structured observation of the patient engaged in an activity is a core skill for the occupational therapist and is concomitant with expertise in task analysis. The therapist may not be able to engage the patient in a formal interview or complete an Assessment of Motor and Process Skills (AMPS). Yet, they may bake cakes with the patient. This kind of assessment is often opportunistic but nevertheless it is rich in data. It is useful to have several carefully analysed activities that can be completed within 30 minutes and initiated when the moment presents itself. The aim is to motivate the patient to undertake a small achievable task, which has a satisfying end product. The task itself will have discrete elements, like written, demonstrated and oral instructions, allowing detailed analysis of the patient's performance. Examples include: assembling a simple wooden construction kit, baking a batch of scones, or printing some personalized notepaper on a printing press or computer. A wealth of information is available through astute observational and listening skills. Table 4.1 provides a useful prompt, although the list is by no means exhaustive.

Table 4.1 Checklist for assessment through observation of activity

- motor skills (fine, gross, coordination)
- communication (verbal and non-verbal, comprehension, language, tone, volume, content, spontaneity)
- sensory (sight, hearing, taste, smell, touch)
- psychosocial (interactions, relationships with other, self-awareness, tolerance, assertiveness, anxiety)
- cognitive abilities (concentration, memory, planning, sequencing, organization, orientation)
- attitude (hostility, acceptance, passivity, aggressiveness, confidence)
- perceptual skills (spatial awareness, figure, ground, etc.)
- process skills (problem-solving, decision-making)
- motivation (intrinsic and extrinsic, level of engagement, stamina)
- insight (needs, behaviour, situation)
- coping strategies (avoidance, overcompensation, withdrawal, substance misuse, self-harm, aggression)

A patient's performance during an activity can reveal subtle changes to their mental state, for example it may show slight deterioration in concentration or fixation on certain topics. For example, one patient in art demonstrated a heightened interest in military paraphernalia. He repeatedly produced war-related work. This provided an early indicator of deterioration in his mental state. In this example, the patient was less guarded in the art group than when seeing the psychiatrist for a formal mental state examination.

Where it is difficult to engage a patient in an activity, the therapist will need to consider why. A suitable choice of activities that are gender and culture appropriate may not have been presented. Or avoidance may signify anxiety and the fear of 'failure'. Many forensic patients have poor literacy skills, which initially can present as difficulty in concentrating. Support, encouragement and careful grading of the activity are indicated in this instance.

Many departments have developed their own tools for checking performance, for example with kitchen assessments, but these may not have been researched and hence may have limited value in measuring progress objectively. Their advantage is that they have been developed to meet specific local needs. Thus, they allow comparison within the setting. For example, they may help to demonstrate a patient's progress in culinary skills and provide a record of the different cooking techniques they have tried. Without proper research though, home-grown tools may fail tests of inter-rater reliability and generalizability.

Interviews are a mainstay of assessment. They provide depth and richer understanding to the assessment. They also help in rapport development. Interviews can have varying degrees of structure and can occur at different stages of the assessment. For example, the initial interview may primarily be a relationship-building exercise whereas a later interview may be specifically undertaken to establish the patient's previous experience in managing household activities of daily living. Finlay (1997) provides a useful guide to interviewing.

Self-rating and standardized tests can be very useful within forensic occupational therapy. Below is a list of those found appropriate and applicable to patients in the Bracton Centre. The purpose and value of each will be highlighted, although the reader may wish to refer to the available publications for more information.

Interest checklist (Rogers 1988)

This provides a useful starting point. The format is non-threatening. It can open up a dialogue including interests pursued prior to admission, the impact of hospitalization, and allows alternative activities to be explored. Prior to administration, it is important to check the patient's level of literacy skills. Where the patient has limited skills, with support, they may wish to read through the form. However, if the patient is embarrassed, fearful or reluctant, the therapist may find it advantageous to read out each item. Items endorsed on the checklist can be used to create an activity of value and significance to the patient. Beware of repeating interest checklists unnecessarily. Check whether one has been completed recently and, if so, use this as a discussion point with the patient, updating information if necessary.

Occupational Self-Assessment – OSA (Baron et al. 2002)

The OSA offers a concise method of eliciting the patient's perceptions of their strengths and needs by exploring performance, habits, roles and volition. The effect of the environment on functioning is considered, which is of particular significance in the forensic setting where both the therapist and patient may have less control of their surroundings. The tool assists the patient to prioritize areas for work. The assessment may be especially valuable when time is of the essence, for example in prison where there may be a rapid turnover of prisoners. The assessment is also useful for patients who may experience some anxiety when faced with an interview situation. The tool is simple to administer and a manual is available. No formal training is required.

Occupational Performance History Interview – OPHI-II (Kielhofner et al. 1998)

The OPHI-II, a semi-structured interview with accompanying rating scales, is based on MoHO. The assessment is flexible and may be completed in stages using all or part of the tool. Detailed information may be derived, including the patient's background, interests, routines, life roles, values and goals and the patient's perceptions of their abilities and needs. The environment and the impact of critical life events are considered. The OPHI-II is a particularly valuable tool which allows a comprehensive picture of the patient's life and their current situation to be gained while aiding the planning of future goals. However, some patients may find the interview situation uncomfortable and intrusive. The assessment tool may at first appear daunting. No formal training is required, but therapists will need to be conversant with MoHO and may wish to observe, or practise, an interview first.

Hampshire Assessment of Living with Others – HALO (Shackleton and Pidcock 1982)

The HALO is a task-based assessment with rating scales to determine levels of independence. The assessment was designed to aid discharge planning, identifying training needs and the level of support required upon discharge. The tool has been useful in the Bracton Centre to screen patients entering a pre-discharge service targeting specific areas of need. HALO encourages collaborative working, particularly between the patient, nursing and occupational therapy staff and is a useful tool to monitor and evaluate the patient's progress. At first glance the tool can appear long and complicated; however, once tried, it is simple and relatively quick to administer and provides comprehensive detail. The manual offers a simple step-by-step guide. No formal training is required.

Assessment of Communication and Interaction Skills – ACIS (Forsyth et al. 1999)

The ACIS is a tool based on observation of communication and interaction skills while engaging in activity within a meaningful social context. The assessment examines 22 skill elements, which fall into three categories: physicality, information exchange and relations. The assessment should be completed in varying social contexts to explore and understand how the environment affects the patient's ability to communicate and interact with others. The assessment requires no formal training, is quick to administer and comes complete with a manual.

Volitional Questionnaire – VQ (Heras et al. 1998)

This is completed while the patient is engaged in activity and allows the therapist to determine the extent of the patient's willingness or ability to engage in three environmental areas: work, leisure and activities of daily living.

Assessment of Motor and Process Skills – AMPS (Fisher 1999)

The AMPS evaluates the underlying motor and process skills needed to complete everyday tasks of varying complexity (instrumental activities of daily living) using structured observation. Five days' formal training is required, which may limit its accessibility to many therapists due to cost implications. Within forensic settings, certain AMPS tasks may provide specific risk management challenges as they require access to sharp implements and other materials. Despite this, clinical experience has demonstrated that the AMPS is an extremely useful outcome measure that can be utilized with a variety of patients.

Guide to implementing assessment

After introducing yourself to the patient and explaining your role within the multiprofessional team, the following sequence should ensure effective, respectful assessment of the patient while not compromising personal safety.

1. **Information gathering** Forensic occupational therapists differ. Some prefer to meet the patient before gathering a detailed forensic history. Their argument is to get to know them before being biased by their offence. Drawing from experience, I recommend reading through all the notes available on the patient, identifying any risk areas or sensitive issues and contacting relevant professionals previously involved. Note any completed assessments to avoid unnecessary repetition; clarity and accuracy of these can be confirmed with the patient. This preparation helps to demonstrate that effort has been made to learn about the patient and their background.

2. **Communication** As a member of the multiprofessional team, occupational therapists have responsibility for communicating and coordinating their work utilizing the Care Programme Approach (CPA) (Department of Health 1999). This entails discussions with the team regarding the proposed occupational therapy assessment. Early on in the patient's admission, several professionals will wish to assess the patient. It is helpful for these assessments to be prioritized in team meetings. This avoids the social worker, occupational therapist, nurse, psychiatrist and psychologist all attempting to assess the patient in one week, usually just prior to a forthcoming CPA meeting!

3. **Timing** It is important to arrange an appointment with the patient at a mutually convenient time. Do not assume that the patient will be able, or wish, to meet you at a time that is convenient only to you. By negotiating times, you are allowing the patient to take some control, exercise planning and decision-making skills, hence promoting a more equal relationship. Consider the information that you already have about the patient. Does the patient suffer extreme drowsiness in the morning? If so will the patient's performance during the assessment be affected and thus not accurately represent the patient's abilities? Consider what the assessment environment will be like at a particular time of the day. For example, if choosing to do a cooking assessment over lunchtime, will the kitchen be too busy? If additional staff support is needed, you may wish to avoid times such as handover or medication.

4. **Preparation** Familiarize yourself with the selected assessment tool or activity. If completing an activity, ensure that all the necessary equipment is available. Once the patient has commenced an activity, it may be difficult to retrieve any additional items as this may result in the patient being left unsupervised.

5. **Choice of room** In addition to selecting a room that is appropriate to the chosen activity and that will optimize performance, consider your own personal safety.
   - Select a room that is central and hence quickly accessible by other staff should you require assistance.
   - Ensure the room is relatively free from clutter and any potential weapons.
   - Choose a reasonably spacious room (a small room may be threatening to the patient; remember the importance of maintaining personal space and how the comfort zone may vary from person to person).
   - Avoid high-stimulus environments or rooms where you are likely to be interrupted, particularly if the patient has difficulties with concentration.

6. **Risk Management** In addition to the above, there are a number of other measures that help to ensure the safety of self and others.
   - Seek a handover from staff prior to your arranged appointment, to elicit whether it is safe and appropriate to proceed with the assessment.
   - Be aware of current care plans and risk assessment.
   - Know where the alarm points are and how to activate them should this be necessary.
   - Position yourself close to the door and ensure that you have a clear escape route.
   - Inform staff of your exact whereabouts and what time you expect to be finished.
   - Remain alert to any subtle changes in the patient's presentation, which may indicate the need to terminate the session and arrange another time to meet.
   - Carry a mobile phone when working in unstaffed areas.
   - Ensure that staff have a contact number should you fail to return within the agreed time.

7. **Inform the patient** Explain what the assessment is for, how the information will be used and who will have access to it. The sharing of information can often be a source of concern for the patient as disclosure of symptoms, or thoughts to harm self or others, can lead to restrictions on leave, observations being imposed or an increase in medication in order to manage risks safely. Clearly, if these strategies are adopted as a direct consequence of the information that has been relayed, trust within the therapeutic relationship may be affected. However, it is vital that all information is shared to maintain the safety of all concerned.

8. **Implementation** Follow any instructions available. This is particularly important if you are implementing a standardized assessment

and wish to maintain the validity of the tool. Give clear instructions to the patient. Establish boundaries by setting and adhering to a time limit on the session. Standardized assessment may remove the personal qualities of communication. The therapist may appear cold and unfeeling if the patient has made some disclosures and the therapist is attempting to continue with the prescribed format of formal assessment tools. A sensitive, flexible and individual approach to assessment is strongly advocated. Acknowledge that the patient may have some performance-related anxieties and that some topic areas may be emotionally difficult for the patient. If you need to take notes, tell the patient that you will be doing so. When taking notes, be sure to maintain an appropriate level of eye contact rather than concentrating solely on your notes! Demonstrate active listening and offer encouraging remarks and gestures. Check the accuracy of what you have written to ensure that you have understood what has been said and have recorded this correctly. Use the patient's words whenever possible.

9. **Share information** Give brief feedback to the team as soon as possible followed by a more detailed summary of the assessment findings. Of equal importance is the feeding back of information to the patient. Brief feedback may be given initially followed by a more comprehensive report. Assessments should be written up as soon as possible to avoid inevitable distortions that occur with lapses in time.

Report writing

When writing up the assessment findings or preparing a progress report, use positive, simple language while remaining professional. The content should be comprehensible to both the patient and to other professionals. Avoid jargon at all costs. Where possible use the patient's words and give examples. Structure your work. You may find it helpful to use the occupational therapy process as a framework for progress reports or to use the selected practice model when writing up specific assessments such as the OPHI-II. Some departments may have developed a pro forma to assist the therapist with report writing. One example is included in Table 4.2 (see below). Refer to the assessment used. State its purpose, the methodology, when and how long it took to administer. Summarize the main findings. Comment upon the observations that were made during the assessment. Clearly identify the patient's strengths and needs including the patient's perception. Always strike a balance between strengths and needs to avoid further damage to self-esteem. Finally, indicate what plans have been devised to address areas of need and what interventions will be used.

Table 4.2 Example structure for an assessment report

[Name of Hospital]

Occupational Therapy [Initial/Review/Specific] Assessment

Name of patient: Date of assessment:
Ward: Date of birth:
Date of admission: Occupational therapist:

Introduction
Clarify the purpose of the report (e.g. to relay assessment findings or to highlight
the progress the patient has made over a fixed period). State the source of
information (e.g. notes, the patient, observation, feedback from other relevant
professionals). Refer to any plans made previously.

Assessment
Name and briefly outline the purpose of the assessment and how it was conducted.
Note any important observations that were made during the assessment.
Summarize areas of need (including the patient's perspective).

Current Occupational Therapy Intervention Plan
Describe the treatment aims and objectives and media used.

Progress
Produce a timetable of the activities that the patient is regularly engaged in. State
whether the patient has been referred to any additional groups/activities. Refer to
the patient's motivation and perceived attitude (consider attendance, level of
engagement and participation). Measure progress against the set objectives.
Highlight skills and needs that have been identified through activity. Consider risk.
Have any concerns been raised: vulnerability/exploitation, practical safety issues,
e.g. road safety, ability to cope with frustration/disappointment, resolution of
conflict, attitude towards/interest in children, alcohol use, etc.

Conclusion
Give an overview of progress made to date and outstanding areas for work.
Proposed occupational therapy intervention plan.
Further areas for assessment. Establish aims and objectives for the next set period.

[Name]:   [Signature]

[Designation]

[Date]

Case Study

Denise is a 25-year-old woman with a psychotic mental illness and a history of substance misuse, arson and assault. When unwell, Denise experiences auditory hallucinations telling her to self-harm or to hurt others. At times, she believes others want to harm her. She secretes potential weapons, usually cutlery, at such times. Denise has on two occasions attempted to stab staff with a fork and has self-harmed by cutting or by swallowing inappropriate items. She discontinued her oral medication when in the community, believing it to be poisoned. Prior to admission, Denise lived at home with her mother and two siblings. Denise has reported sexual abuse within the family. Through observation, the records available and feedback from other professionals a number of needs were identified, which will be illustrated using MoHO as a framework.

Volition

Denise's interests appeared to centre around the family and were generally initiated by family members. Very few were activities that she could pursue alone and hence encouraged dependence upon others. She appeared to lack confidence in her abilities, relying upon others to carry out tasks for her, which limited the development of her own skills. Denise valued her family, her main goal being to return to live with them – a goal not shared by the team. Other values included her appearance.

Habituation

When removed from the context of her family, Denise appeared to have some difficulty in adjusting to new routines and adopting other life roles, including the formation of relationships with both staff and peers. She lacked awareness of others' needs and was vulnerable to exploitation, particularly by male patients. Contact with her family was minimal due to Denise's distance from the family home. Owing to these factors, Denise spent long periods asleep in her bedroom.

Performance

Denise's skills in a number of areas appeared poor due to her reliance upon others and the limited opportunities that had been afforded her in the community. Areas of need included: personal and domestic activities of daily living, particularly personal hygiene, diet and cooking, literacy and numeracy, interpersonal skills and community living skills (public transport, shopping, awareness and use of community facilities).

OT involvement

Denise was asked to complete an interest checklist to stimulate discussion about activities that she might like to choose from and experiment with. This encouraged her to make choices and to accept a degree of responsibility for herself. Denise appeared willing to engage although she remained quiet, responding only to questions. Her responses were mostly monosyllabic.

The activity she chose was cooking, and this was undertaken away from the kitchen to safely manage the potential risks involved. As Denise's access to both sharps and the kitchen was restricted the recipe selected required few utensils and limited use of appliances. The main aims of the activity were to:

* promote the therapeutic relationship
* encourage interactions with others
* provide Denise with a sense of achievement through successful completion of an activity
* begin assessment of Denise's functional skills.

A developmental approach was used, with the therapist working alongside Denise, sharing tasks and providing information as necessary. Denise successfully produced favourable results, which she shared with other patients and staff on the ward, receiving much praise and encouragement. The sessions highlighted a number of strengths and needs. Written reports of Denise's progress were made available to her, and she was actively encouraged to comment upon her performance. After several more individual sessions, Denise began to experiment with other activities such as adult education and use of the gym, relying less on the therapist for support and direction. Her awareness of others increased, and she appeared more confident in her interactions, establishing a close working relationship with other members of the multiprofessional team. Gradually, Denise began working alongside, and then with, other patients.

To ascertain Denise's perception of her needs, the OSA was administered. This was chosen because the tool is quick and easy to administer. This was important, as Denise's concentration was impaired. She experienced particular difficulties when faced with formal situations, which provoked anxiety within her. Also the OSA offered a structure for Denise to consider her own values and needs and assisted her in planning and prioritizing her own goals. Denise was able to identify a number of areas that she wished to improve and prioritized these in order of importance. Top of her list was leaving hospital. Identification of this goal assisted the therapist and Denise to negotiate intervention plans. Denise recognized that she needed help with a number of areas including shopping, budgeting, menu planning and cooking – all essential skills for successful discharge. The HALO was selected as a tool to obtain a baseline of Denise's daily living skills. The intervention plan focused on the areas of need highlighted, with priority areas being addressed first. After further intervention, the HALO was repeated to measure objectively the progress made.

Conclusion

This chapter has explored the reasons for assessment and provides practical information regarding the selection, planning and implementation of assessment methods. A number of tools have been reviewed and the importance of using observation and listening skills highlighted. A coordinated team approach to assessment has been emphasized together with the encouragement of active patient involvement. Consideration has been given to risk and management strategies that can be adopted to enable a safe working environment. Finally, guidelines have been offered to assist report writing and information-sharing with both the patient and the clinical team.

References

Baron K, Kielhofner G, Iyenger A, Goldhammer V and Wolenski J (2002) The Occupational Self-Assessment – Version 2.0. Chicago: University of Illinois.

Buchan T (2002) The impact of language and culture when administering the assessment of motor and process skills: A case study. British Journal of Therapy and Rehabilitation 65(8) 371–373.

College of Occupational Therapists (1995) Standards, Policies and Procedures: Guidelines for Occupational Therapy Services in Mental Health, 110A (January). London: College of Occupational Therapists.

Department of Health (1998) National Service Framework for Mental Health. London: Department of Health.

Department of Health (1999) Effective Care Coordination in Mental Health Services: Modernising the Care Programme Approach. London: Department of Health.

Finlay L (1997) The Practice of Psychosocial Occupational Therapy (2nd edition). Cheltenham: Stanley Thornes.

Fisher A (1999) Assessment of Motor and Process Skills (3rd edition). Fort Collins, Colorado: Three Star Press.

Forsyth K, Lai J-S and Kielhofner G (1999) The assessment of communication and interaction skills (ACIS): Measurement properties. British Journal of Occupational Therapy 62(2) 69–74.

Fuller J and Cowan J (1999) Risk assessment in a multi-disciplinary forensic setting: Clinical judgement revisited. Journal of Forensic Psychiatry 10(2) 276–289.

Hagedorn R (1995) Occupational Therapy Perspectives and Processes. Edinburgh: Churchill Livingstone.

Heras C, Geist R and Kielhofner G (1998) The Volitional Questionnaire (VQ). Chicago: University of Illinois.

Kielhofner G (1997) The Conceptual Foundations of Occupational Therapy (2nd edition). Philadelphia: F. A. Davis Company.

Kielhofner G, Mallinson T, Crawford C, Nowak M, Rigby M, Henry A and Walens D (1998) The Occupational Performance History Interview – Version 2.0. Chicago: University of Illinois.

Law M, Steinwender S and Leclair L (1998) Occupation, Health and Well-being. Canadian Journal of Occupational Therapy 65(2) 81–91.

McAdam K, Thomas W and Chard G (2001) The assessment of motor and process skills: An evaluation of the impact of training on service delivery. British Journal of Occupational Therapy 64(7) 357–363.

Rogers J (1988) The NPI Interest Checklist. In: Mental Health Assessment in Occupational Therapy, Hemphill B (ed.). Thorofare NJ: Slack.

Seally C (1999) Clinical governance: An information guide for occupational therapists. British Journal of Occupational Therapy 62(6) 263–268.

Shackleton M and Pidcock B (1982) Hampshire Assessment for Living with Others. Hampshire: Social Services Department of Hampshire County Council.

Snowden P (1997) Practical aspects of clinical risk assessment and management. British Journal of Psychiatry 170(32) 32–34.

Vaughan G and Done D (2000) Recent research relevant to discharge planning from medium secure psychiatric units: Re-examining the literature. Journal of Forensic Psychiatry 11(2) 372–389.

Wilson M (1987) Occupational Therapy in Long-term Psychiatry (2nd edition). Edinburgh: Churchill Livingstone.

CHAPTER 5

Programme planning

DEBORAH ALRED

Introduction

The planning and co-ordination of a comprehensive therapy and rehabilitation programme is one of the key roles of the forensic occupational therapist. This chapter considers the development of purposeful inpatient programmes within forensic settings. It begins with a view of the client group, identifying some of the considerations that need to be addressed in terms of the programme and moves on to a review of some of the types of groups that contribute to the overall programme. Finally staff development issues involved with planning and sustaining a full and balanced programme are discussed. I present these thoughts as a starting point; they have come from my experience and from the experience of other head occupational therapists working within similar settings.

Regional secure units have been established with a high staff:patient ratio in the expectation that this will produce greater therapeutic efficacy and greater security (Stone et al. 2000). Occupational therapists, with their understanding of how activity can be adapted and used to meet specific therapeutic needs, are in an ideal position to facilitate therapeutic endeavour. This includes consideration of the environment, the routine and the activities carried out. I work in medium and low secure units as well as a hostel; where the occupational therapy areas are incorporated into the units, there is no separate department. As a result of this, the occupational therapy programme is integrated into the running of the unit. Throughout this chapter, I shall mainly be referring to occupational therapy and nursing staff, as they are the two largest staff groups that work together to affect the therapeutic life on our unit.

The client group

The admission criteria for this client group is based on their security needs coupled with their mental disorder. This results in a client group admitted with a range of presentations and needs. If they have been admitted via court diversion, they may be in the middle of an acute psychotic episode. If from a high secure unit like Broadmoor, Rampton, Ashworth or Carstairs, they are potentially stable and ready for continued rehabilitation. Residents often present with a dual diagnosis and a range of developmental, mental health and substance misuse needs. If residents have an ongoing court case, their attention may be directed towards preparation for this. This can be coupled with a reluctance to engage in any aspect of unit life because of their expectation of imminent release.

Staff recognize and have elected to spend their working day in the presence of violent and dangerous people, but the residents have not; they are compelled to be there. They can be nervous of other residents and reluctant to spend more time with them than necessary. They may have difficulty coping with the intrusive and demanding behaviour of others on the unit, resulting in them staying in their rooms to avoid other residents or conflict. Forensic patients who have been admitted under section are subject to different release criteria than other client groups. This can lead to extended hospital stays and can cause frustration and disappointment if discharge is delayed. This may result in a re-emergence of symptoms or a feeling of resentment towards the therapist if the resident sees the therapist as being impotent in giving assistance (Lloyd 1995). In my service the average length of stay is seven months in the medium secure unit, and four years in the low secure unit.

All this means that on the unit at any one time you will be presented with a group of residents with a wide range of skills, abilities and needs. Some will be motivated and engaged in the programme. Others will be unwilling to become engaged in anything that involves them with the unit. This range of needs presents a considerable challenge to the occupational therapists when identifying priorities for the programme.

Programme development has many meanings. In this chapter, it is referring both to the planning, coordination and implementation of a full range of activities as well as the way services can be coordinated to make this happen. MacDonald (1978 p.274) neatly describes the general aims of a programme for long-stay patients as 'Remotivation, Resocialisation, Retraining and Resettlement'. This relates well to what we are trying to achieve within a forensic setting. With the forensic client group in mind, a multilevel group programme providing a range of opportunities and meeting a range of therapeutic goals is recommended.

Unit community activities

These are general recreational and diversionary activities around the unit. They are designed to provide a variety of opportunities for individuals to participate in activities, the goal being to promote residents' mental and social well-being (Ryan 1993). The occupational may not facilitate all these activities but have a role with their coordination and supporting ward staff in developing them. This may include providing practical support like ingredients for cooking sessions, training staff in techniques and providing supervision. It also includes generating a positive creative environment and using information from residents as a starting point for the activities allowing each ward to develop its own internal culture. The occupational therapist's openness to the ideas and interests of the residents and understanding about how to put them into practice in a safe and realistic way can help to facilitate the programme and involve both residents and staff. In our rehabilitation unit, outings and cooking have been consistently the most requested activities, and this is reflected in the programme.

We have recently bought some bicycles to facilitate individual and group outings. Safety considerations are addressed by establishing clear guidelines about who can have access to the bikes as well as ensuring safety equipment is available. The use of a formal assessment of competency on the bikes engenders a sense of responsibility and reinforces road sense. Ward staff interested in facilitating activities who cannot commit themselves to regular weekly groups, owing to ward commitments and varying shifts, run ad hoc practical sessions with the residents, ensuring the bicycles are well maintained. The bicycles allow for the development of individual rehabilitation programmes. Residents have used the cycles to travel to work rehabilitation centres and to the shops for buying ingredients. Likewise, ward staff have used them to take advantage of good days by taking a group out. They provide the physical activity for individuals who may be reluctant to participate in sport. These principles of identifying themes or activities and analysing them ensure clear protocols and safety procedures. This facilitates staff involvement and can be applied to a range of projects on the ward.

A consistent activity programme provides a stable predictable structure that forms the bedrock of an activity-based therapeutic programme. It provides an opportunity for residents to build relationships and develop a sense of community. A successful activity programme involves much more than the planning and carrying out of activities. It must also include the 'creation of an atmosphere that offers decision making opportunities and promotes independence and an atmosphere where residents are offered encouragement and support but are never coerced or forced to participate. These are very important motivational factors' (Ryan 1993 p.198).

Task activities

Within the forensic environment, occupational therapists are rediscovering their core skills. Occupational therapy task interventions may be incorporated into an activity programme, but they will have very different aims from recreational activities. Analysis of the activity being carried out and observation of the resident's performance in an individual or group setting allows the occupational therapist to focus on the 'person as doer' and 'enable problems and needs to be understood and treatment goals to be set' (Hagedorn 1997 p.26). Through facilitation and monitoring of individuals within an activity framework the occupational therapist can assess all aspects of performance skills and use this information to plan other aspects of the programme.

Psycho-education programme

When residents have the concentration and ability to benefit from more structured and focused interventions, this is the time to involve them in group work developed to address specific problems. Psycho-educational groups are designed to look at and develop specific coping skills (Eaton 2002). They make use of cognitive and behavioural techniques. They can incorporate learning about the specific mental health conditions and the practice of techniques to address symptoms. Groups such as anxiety or anger management give the resident valuable information about the general processes involved and strategies that they can relate to their own situation and put into practice in the ward environment. In terms of anxiety management, residents can begin to use techniques for a stressful situation, such as attending ward round, by talking it through in the group before the event and feeding back how they got on. This kind of exercise builds knowledge and confidence in the techniques. Various members of the team facilitate these groups, this increases the experience and perspectives brought to the groups. The residents also benefit by seeing professionals in a different setting.

Supportive group work

As residents become more confident in these cognitive behavioural techniques, work designed to integrate them into a group, and address issues more personal to them, can be developed in the context of supportive group work. One example from our service is the 'Moving on Group', a pre-discharge group that allows residents to prepare for discharge by sharing any feelings and anxieties. It provides a forum for discussion and support. Again, multidisciplinary facilitation of the groups is ideal.

Similarly, at any stage in an individual's stay the use of non-verbal creative therapies, such as art and music therapy facilitated by qualified creative therapists and jointly run by unit staff, can offer a safe forum for the expression and the exploration of feelings.

Adult education

The stay in a residential setting can provide the most stable environment some residents have experienced for a long time. This allows an opportunity for adult learning to occur. Developing relationships with staff in local adult learning establishments permits supported access to a range of courses. Colleges may also be willing to provide funding for teachers to undertake basic adult learning within the secure environment. However, their minimum-numbers criteria can be unrealistic. Some forensic units fund adult education teachers to enable smaller classes to address this issue. Local Education Authorities increasingly are looking at strategies to include all in education. They are willing to work in partnership to identify and run relevant courses and support residents in attending open courses. Vocational classes such as painting and decorating have provided a useful link to help individuals to develop social networks and a bridge to the outside world.

Work rehabilitation

'Not only does work provide a sense of worth and value for the individual but it also provides a source of social contacts which helps provide a normalising social network' (Lloyd 1995 p.121). Residents need to develop experience in all aspects of work skills, including completing application forms, interview techniques and work discipline. The development of work opportunities allows individuals to gain experience in a supportive environment geared towards their individual needs. For a work programme to be progressive, it must involve close liaison with a number of agencies and other services that specialize in work experience and placement. Work experience can be developed in-house with residents taking on specific job skills such as decorating or gardening, some units have set up NVQ courses aligned with these placements. Initially, residents will participate in work by taking on jobs to supplement their income, but the responsibility that they have, for example turning up on time, can incrementally develop the disciplines necessary for progressing further.

Developing links with local work rehabilitation projects provides worthwhile access to specialist facilities. We have set up a project whereby nursing and occupational therapy staff accompany residents to a local work rehabilitation centre for a total of four sessions a week. The staff involved spent time thinking through systems of communication and the roles each would take while at the centre. It was considered important that the forensic staff took on meaningful roles within the centre in order to foster continued skill sharing as well as providing a low-key escort. This has been a valuable service to residents as they required a consistent work routine, and it has also provided experience for residents who may be referred to similar centres in their local area on discharge.

Currently, we have residents with high levels of skill and who are potentially capable of employment in the open market; however, work needs to be done to provide opportunities to support this. Ruth Garner (1995) describes a successful project, which linked Reaside, a medium secure unit, with Birmingham City Training Agents. This enabled the secure unit to draw on the training agency's expertise in developing employment skills. Organization of jobs, monitoring performance, organizing payments, making the experience relevant to individual needs and feeding back progress to the wider team require considerable staff time and effort. Ideally, dedicated staff would be involved, as they can continue to develop specialist expertise. This is not always practical in smaller units.

Establishing relationships with outside agencies in relation to education and work opportunities allows occupational therapists to address some of the fears and stigma that surround forensic clients. It can take time for communication systems to be developed and to organize safe risk-assessed interventions. On occasion this has meant that the resident, for whom the system was originally set up has been discharged or become ill and unable to participate. Although this can be demoralizing, the effort is not wasted because, once relationships with other agencies have been established, they can be maintained for future residents.

Getting the balance

When developing programmes, it is important to be realistic about what can be achieved. It is unlikely that all residents will be involved with all activities, and the range of clinical presentations means that decisions have to be made. It is up to occupational therapists through detailed assessment and close collaboration, with both the resident and the care team, to develop a programme that will suit the resident's immediate needs. Likewise, it is essential to undertake regular reviews to ensure that the programme is meeting identified needs and is progressive.

I have presented these types of groups in a linear way; however, each may be suitable for individuals at any one time in the context of their own progression. 'All programmes need to be realistic and build into them flexibility to take into account possible relapses in mental health, pace of learning, medication, confidence, previous experience, and restrictions' (Garner 1995 p.3). Considering the average length of stay of residents, it can be effective to organize the group work into 10-week blocks with breaks of diverting activities in between. This has worked well in some units. This allows space for a review of the groups and punctuates the year, giving residents opportunities for time off and 'holidays'. It also allows for seasonal activities to be added to the programme at appropriate moments, for example providing craft groups leading up to the Christmas period as residents make presents for friends and family.

Encouraging staff

The provision of a dynamic and exciting programme is a truly multiprofessional endeavour, and effort must be put into facilitating staff involvement and coordination. This includes ensuring the support of managers to release staff, enabling them to participate in the group programme. Not only do they need structured time within their working day to facilitate groups but also time is needed to prepare and review the interventions. Commitment from the whole team is necessary to identify and address barriers to multidisciplinary working. This can be challenging for all involved, particularly in the context of the range of demands of the unit, but good professional skills should ensure it is done in a positive way.

Multidisciplinary involvement in activity groups requires considerable effort, coordination and education. In a forensic setting this is particularly so because of the higher numbers of staff involved; however, it 'reaps the benefits of increased status of groups and support in running them' (Fairbairn 2000 p.292). It is worth spending time with individual members of staff to identify their interest in involvement with the programme and educating them about the purpose of the programme within the unit. We have recently initiated a joint nursing and occupational therapy induction, which is proving to be a good introduction for all new staff entering the unit. Each new staff member spends a week with the complementary staff group. Occupational therapy staff gain an insight into how the ward as a whole operates, and nursing staff learn some of the principles of the activity programme and how they can become involved.

Setting up systems to support staff development within groups helps to facilitate a learning culture and promotes expertise throughout the wider team. Multidisciplinary meetings like the group development forum, chaired by a psychologist, provide a space where all disciplines that want to carry out group work come together to discuss their proposals and coordinate the groups. This includes practical issues such as location and times of groups as well as ensuring the group programme is complementary. It also provides a space for feedback and planning of future developments and a forum where standards for the groups can be agreed and any issues affecting group work can be discussed. In this way, the group programme for the service is responsive to identified resident need. For example, the residents reported that they needed to feel more comfortable being in a group before they could benefit from some of the psycho-educational or supportive group work. In response, a group was established to address this need.

Education and engagement of the team in the therapy programme is crucial to its success. Inclusion of the individual's therapy and activity plan within the care plan sets the therapy in the context of the rest of the treatment regime. Feedback and discussion about each resident's participation in activity, in the ward round, reinforces its place within the resident's overall treatment plan and provides valuable information to the multidisciplinary team. Ward staff need to be familiar with an individual's activity plan to ensure that it is considered within the practical running of the ward, for example booking other appointments around it. Informal discussion about this programme involves all staff and again provides support to the programme. If you find you are spending more time talking about what you are planning to do than actually doing it, you are probably getting the balance right. This will be reflected in the smooth running of the group and the reinforcement of staff in assisting with motivating residents to attend and then asking them about it afterwards.

An open and inclusive approach to the development of groups allows individual staff members to be supported as their confidence increases and their skills advance. Psycho-educational or support groups have been successfully facilitated by three facilitators, two of whom may be more experienced while one takes on a learning or observational role. As well as contributing to observations about the development of the group, skills are learned and practised in a safe context. This system has the additional advantage of ensuring that the group will continue if one facilitator is unable to attend. This flexibility is particularly important when supporting the involvement of nursing staff in groups who may be asked to cover staff shortages or be called back to the ward if it is disturbed. After much experimentation, we have found that, in order to promote ward staff involvement, taking them off numbers and involving them in a nine-to-five shift once a week promotes consistent group involvement.

When considering activities, the interests and knowledge of staff can be harnessed and adapted to suit the resident's needs. For example, we have popular and successful car maintenance and photography groups. These are run by combining the task skills of the nursing staff and the group planning expertise of occupational therapists. Establishing small multidisciplinary groups to research and set up specialist groups increases the skills base of the team. It also ensures that the groups developed are based on best practice and delivered in a way that is right for the staff and based on the needs of the residents. Some of the advantages of working in a small speciality such as forensic psychiatry are the increased communication and opportunity for sharing best practice, and learning from the expertise of others working in similar areas. For example, Glen Thomas, a clinical nurse specialist at Rampton Hospital, has developed a group for substance misuse for patients in a high secure setting. He has generously provided support and shared his material so that it can be used in our setting.

Conclusion

A consistent activity programme provides a stable and predictable foundation, the bedrock on which forensic occupational therapy occurs. The provision of a dynamic, successful and exciting programme demands a truly multiprofessional endeavour. In this chapter, I have reviewed some of the staffing and organizational issues involved with the development of a therapy programme within medium and low secure units. Possible strategies have been identified to promote multidisciplinary involvement in the programme and this chapter has given a picture of some of the types of group and intervention that work together to produce a comprehensive programme.

References

Eaton P (2002) Psychoeducation in acute mental health settings: Is there a role for occupational therapists? British Journal of Occupational Therapy 65(7) 321–326.

Fairbairn C (2000) Psychiatric rehabilitation units: How can occupational therapists help them into the new millennium? British Journal of Occupational Therapy 63(6) 291–293.

Garner R (1995) Prevocational training within a secure environment: A programme designed to enable the forensic patient to prepare for mainstream opportunities. British Journal of Occupational Therapy 58(1) 2–6.

Hagedorn R (1997) Foundations for Practice in Occupational Therapy (2nd edition). Edinburgh: Churchill Livingstone.

Lloyd C (1995) Forensic Psychiatry for Health Professionals. London: Chapman and Hall.

MacDonald E (1978) Occupational Therapy in Rehabilitation (4th edition). Aberdeen: Baillière Tindall.

Ryan S (1993) Practice Issues in Occupational Therapy, Intraprofessional Team Building. Thorofare NJ: Slack.

Stone J, Roberts M, O'Grady J and Taylor A with O'Shea K (2000) Faulk's Basic Forensic Psychiatry (3rd edition). Oxford: Blackwell Science.

CHAPTER 6

Everyone is an artist

MARK SPYBEY AND PHIL MORGAN

Introduction

Occupational therapists working in mental health have been historically associated with using creative activities as a treatment medium. Have you ever thought why occupational therapists use activities that promote creativity, or questioned whether these activities are relevant in a forensic psychiatric setting? What benefit can painting a picture or writing a song have for our clients?

Most of our clients have experienced significant distress in their lives. Their mental health problems often started at an early age. They frequently suffer from both the positive and negative symptoms of mental illness or are ravaged by years of substance misuse. They have engaged in crimes that are often serious and significant. They come from 'troubled', predominantly working-class, backgrounds. It seems somewhat ironic to use the term 'working class', because many of our clients will not have had the opportunity to work legitimately. They will probably have served time in various institutions that accidentally, or in actuality, seek to diminish their ability to engage in occupations. Our clients are often culturally impoverished, understimulated and invariably confined. Whatever appreciation they may have had of their skills and abilities therefore may have been eroded.

The central part of the occupational therapist's role is to provide clients with opportunities to rediscover, develop and/or maintain their skills, interests and goals. This can be done in a variety of positive and meaningful ways, one of which is through the use of creative activities.

Definitions of creativity tend to focus on the individual's ability to generate or recognize new ideas, alternatives or possibilities in an attempt to solve problems (Franken 2001). Clinicians and especially creative therapists have suggested that by being creative we learn more about ourselves, other people and the world we inhabit (Gordon 1983).

In 1989, the Council of Europe acknowledged the role that creative activities can play in the rehabilitation of offenders in their document

Education in Prisons (Council of Europe 1989). This document suggests that through engagement in creative activity the individual can make the transition from offender to citizen by developing a positive sense of self. Economic well-being can result from the development of skills that can help individuals find work. In addition, the individual can improve the way they make judgements, self-reflect and engage socially. This chapter will highlight how occupational therapists can help their clients, through the use of creative activity, to promote and develop self-efficacy skills and thus facilitate their road to recovery.

Everyone is an artist

The artist has, to a certain extent, occupied a position of privilege within society. From Michelangelo to Damien Hirst, artists have been offered the support of benefactors and have, perhaps arguably, enjoyed the enviable position of having their observations (which have often been provocative) both listened to and, to a certain extent, respected. Mentally ill people and offenders can be creative and, although they have not been regarded as 'gatekeepers' of the arts in the same way as artists, art critics or art students have, it is important to promote the idea that the arts are open to all and are both socially and culturally meaningful.

Creative expression is central to every culture's sense of identity. Art is involved in shaping and influencing social and political movements. For example, the writer and former dissident Václav Havel is now the President of the Czech Republic. The 'artists' of the Situationist Internationale inspired events that led to the Paris riots of 1968, which very nearly led to the demise of the French Government. Countless artists across the world have been imprisoned or pilloried for their beliefs.

Appreciation of the aesthetic is intrinsically linked to people's everyday lives whether it is through watching television, cooking or listening to music. People constantly make choices about what they like or dislike. It was the German artist Joseph Beuys (1921–1986) who proclaimed, in a television documentary, with understated eloquence 'everyone is an artist' (1988). He also said:

> The essential definition of a human being is that of 'artist'. All other definitions of the word 'art' lead back to the idea that there are artists and non-artists, of people who can do something and others who can't.

Actor and dramatist Steven Berkoff (1991) wrote in a letter to one of the authors:

> I believe the idea that everyone is an artist is a paramount truth and something that has been denied to most people who follow the very middle-class precept that only certain types of people are privileged to call themselves this. Consequently, we have a very dull art.

It is interesting to reflect that artists' lifestyles (as with our clients) are often seen to conflict with societal norms. According to Felix Post (1994), artists are more likely to suffer with various pathological personality traits, as well as tendencies towards depression and alcoholism. He suggests these characteristics are related to, or possibly caused by, some kind of valuable creativity. What is also interesting is the link between risk taking and creativity; according to the jazz musician and composer Benny Golson (cited in Goleman et al. 1993), creative people are committed to the notion of taking risks. He differentiates between those who follow the path of light (what is known) as opposed to those who rely on their innate drive to be creative and, as a consequence, create their own path, veering into the darkness of the unknown.

All of our clients do, or have, engaged in risky behaviours, and part of our role is to help our clients manage their behaviours and minimize these risks. Through engagement in creative activity, clients are able to explore their own creativity and take risks in a controlled and safe way.

Engagement in creative activity or creative therapy

Are occupational therapists entitled to use creative activities as part of their therapeutic media or should this be the remit only of the creative therapists (such as art, music, dance and drama therapists) whose training is primarily focused on the dynamic use of creative media?

We would argue that there is a role for both professional groups to work with creative techniques and that the difference is in the focus of the treatment process. Occupational therapy should not be preoccupied with interpreting the content of, or exploring the client's inner feelings experienced through, their client's art. The therapeutic concern in occupational therapy is in the doing itself. Art is an occupational form that is present in all cultures and encompasses both leisure and productive aspects. The idea that the therapeutic value is 'in the doing' is reflected in the ideas of the artist and writer Mary Barnes (1923-2001), who suffered with mental illness for many years. Mary suggested that art should be accepted for what it is as opposed to how it may be analysed (Barnes and Scott 1989).

The creative process

It is easy to say that the therapeutic process is in the doing, but how can we help our clients 'do' art? In addressing this, it is important to explore the different stages of the creative process and how they relate to occupational therapy. Goleman et al. (1993) identify that it was the French mathematician Jules Henri Poincaré (1854-1912) who first articulated these stages, but these observations have been repeated by numerous theorists. The four main stages are:

1. Preparation

When we engage in creative activity, we encourage a state of active preparation. We become immersed in the activity and juxtapose a variety of elements (the pen, the paper, the canvas, the brush, the clay, the table, the sticky-back plastic, the empty bottle of detergent) and seek to make some kind of connection between them.

During this stage, we may rely on our ability to arrive at mundane solutions. For example, the empty bottle of detergent is better off being thrown away instead of being transformed into a space rocket or a handy pencil holder for your favourite uncle. Alternatively, we may trust the voice of the inner sceptic (if I do something unfamiliar, people will think I am foolish) or become frustrated at our apparent lack of progress.

We are continually presented with clients who successfully manage to talk themselves out of engaging in creative activity. Ever heard something like this? 'I can't paint, I was told at school that I can't paint.' Similarly, I'm sure that we have all worked with clients who become easily frustrated by some activities or are deemed to have cognitive deficits or poor motivation. After all, there are many factors that contribute to engagement problems. Perhaps the most potent is avoidance. The 'I'm not even going to try' trap that regrettably both therapists and their clients can fall into. It is a kind of institutional choicelessness or uninspired negativism.

It is our role as occupational therapists to attempt to counteract this and, in some ways, it is the most difficult step. We must draw upon our knowledge of our clients in order to provide a stimulus, or volitional hook, of things that they are interested in, or may have been interested in in the past. It is then our role to provide opportunities, give unconditional positive regard and supply the materials to enable clients to engage in the preparatory stage.

2. Incubation

Second, we incubate ideas. We passively digest the information that we have gathered. It is presumed that much of this goes on outside of one's focused awareness. This is a neuro-psychological process and has been identified as such by Sperry, Gazzingen and Bogen (cited in Zdenek 1985). They have been able to illustrate the differences between the way the right and left sides of the brain work and posit that certain processes are more typically associated with the right brain than the left. Hoppe (cited in Zdenek 1985) suggested that by stimulating the right side of the brain, we are able to develop imaginative ability.

Put simply, a left-brain response to the prospect of engagement in creative activity is to talk oneself out of doing it or to simply see the empty detergent bottle as an empty bottle of detergent. The right-side approach is dynamic in the sense that it allows for the possibility of creative engage-ment, but with no guarantee of successful outcome. The empty detergent bottle may become part of a Martian landscape or, indeed, it may not. Artists refer to this as 'the empty canvas' syndrome, the canvas being both the potential masterpiece and the disaster. So we use activities that stimu-late the right brain into exploring new possibilities and developing new insights. Amabile (1983) asserts that the essence of creative engagement is the drive to explore, to develop new ways of overcoming problems.

Having prepared for, and successfully engaged in, creative activity it is now our responsibility to ensure that the client feels able to stay with the activity. We do so by discussing the ideas generated by the work, providing access to additional materials and equipment, helping clients foster new and novel approaches and to promote increased awareness of problem-solving. Fundamentally linked to this is the drive to take risks. No matter how small, a risk is still a risk. Sustained engagement in the activity itself requires that risks are taken, and it is our role to provide the possibility for clients to take graded risks in a safe and supported manner.

3. Illumination

The third phase of the creative process is the moment of illumination. It is the moment where we suddenly feel a rush of satisfaction or achievement. The answer appears to you as if from nowhere. Artists often refer to this moment as 'the creative high'. It is important to note that this moment can-not happen without the realization of the preparatory and incubative stages. In this stage the occupational therapist can provide the reinforcement of the value of the 'creative high' and support their clients to maintain their volition to see the project into transformation stage and thus to completion.

4. Transformation

Finally, we transform our experience into action. Rather than being a moment of transitory insight, we regard the benefits obtained as being useful. Many of our clients have difficulty accepting that they have posi-tive attributes or skills of worth, a kind of learned worthlessness if you like. There is a general acknowledgement that social processes play a major role in the recognition of creativity (Amabile 1983). Many of our clients have considerable problems relating to others and may come from dysfunctional families. Consequently, there may be intense social pres-sure exerted upon them to conform to roles and behaviours that do not militate in favour of change or growth. When the task is completed, we should encourage clients to reflect on the process and to focus on how problems were solved and risks were taken. It is also of benefit to discuss how these thoughts may be generalized.

It is important to note that throughout the stages of this process, different clients will need different levels of support, and activities will need to be graded accordingly.

Jack's story

Jack has spent the past eight years in prison and a medium secure unit. Jack has a history of psychosis, self-harm and substance abuse. Prior to his arrest and subsequent transfer to hospital, he would spend his days drinking, taking drugs and engaging in petty crime, occasionally working for short periods of time doing menial work.

Jack was notoriously difficult to engage. Whenever Jack appeared close to engaging he would abscond, get drunk or take drugs. A new occupational therapist on the ward made contact with Jack not by asking to assess him formally but by sitting and talking with him as often as he could in the clients' lounge. It transpired that when Jack was younger he used to make models out of scrap paper and cardboard. Jack stated that he had wanted to do this again but had been told that he would have to join an art group to be able to get the materials. Jack was not interested in this as he perceived his model making as something personal and wished to do it in his room. The occupational therapist then advocated for Jack in the ward round and negotiated that Jack could have the materials he needed to make the models in his room. In advocating for Jack, the occupational therapist built up a trusting relationship and Jack became increasingly at ease talking about his model making. The occupational therapist and Jack began community trips together visiting transport museums and model shops to develop his interest.

Jack began making small and intricate models of cars and ships in his room. He would work from no plans but would have clear ideas of how they were going to look. On completion, he demonstrated a sense of pride and was given positive feedback. He became increasingly keen to invite staff and his peers into his room to show his work. He developed his interest by making small pieces of furniture from papier mâché that were both aesthetic and functional. He would give these as gifts to his peers.

Jack became more receptive to new ideas and began to reflect on his previous lifestyle. He grew in confidence from the positive feedback that he began to receive both from staff and peers. With support from the occupational therapist, he began to contemplate going to college to study carpentry.

Obviously, not all of our clients will make such dramatic progress, but this case study does demonstrate that when people engage in creative activity they can make small changes by improving their performance skills, quality of life and self-esteem.

Conclusion

The rehabilitative process within forensic psychiatry is rarely a predictable or logical one. While the creative process is not a mechanistic one, it does suggest a structure that may enable us to understand how we engage clients in such activity. In our work, we have to provide opportunities for success and failure. We have to encourage legitimate risk taking. We can do so through engagement in creative activity because it is the activity itself that requires the participant to take risks, even if, as in the case of Jack and his model making, the risks are relatively low. Creative engagement is not a mystical or magical process. It is an innate volitional drive and it is one that we all maintain, regardless of our educational, social or cultural background and regardless of our relative strengths and needs.

Occupational therapists should not shirk from providing arts activities 'for their own sake'. Activities could cover a multitude of areas such as painting, drawing, sculpture, writing, drama, dance, movement, mime, music, pottery, photography, furniture making, cookery, needlecraft, basket making (yes, even basket making) and computer-aided design and video making.

By preparing and then facilitating effective engagement in creative activity, we set up options or problems that need to be addressed. By definition, we need to trust implicitly the clients' ability to think imaginatively and that, consequently, there is therapeutic benefit to be gained from being creative.

References

Amabile T (1983) The Social Psychology of Creativity. New York: Springer-Verlag.

Barnes M and Scott H (1989) Something Sacred: Conversations, Writings, Paintings. London: Free Association Books.

Berkoff S (1991) Personal communication to Mark Spybey.

Beuys J (1988) State of the Art, BBC Television Documentary. London: British Broadcasting Corporation.

Council of Europe (1989) Education in Prisons. Luxembourg: Council of Europe.

Franken R (2001) Human Motivation. New York: Brooks Cole.

Goleman D, Raufman P and Ray M (1993) The Creative Spirit. New York: Plume.

Gordon R (1983) The creative process: self-expression and self-transcendence. In: Creative Therapy, Jennings S (ed.). Banbury: Kemble Press.

Post F (1994) Creativity and Psychopathology: A study of 291 world famous men. British Journal of Psychiatry 165(2) 22–34.

Zdenek M (1985) The Right-brain Experience. London: Corgi Books.

CHAPTER 7

Cognitive behavioural group work within forensic occupational therapy

REBECCA KELLY

Introduction

Group work is a treatment medium commonly used by occupational therapists as a way of providing therapy in a psychosocial setting. Groups can be used to offer a wide range of treatments from task-based activity through to social development and communication skills. Groups can effectively focus on the development of the individual within the context of a social environment.

Forensic patients often have lifelong difficulties establishing cooperative relationships, and it is for this reason that the Oxford Clinic (medium security) focuses on the importance of group work. Within the ward environment, it is important to develop some sense of social belonging. I have seen many instances where patients have been completely withdrawn or extremely demanding if their own needs are not met immediately. They can be unaware of the needs of others unless they coincide with their own. On a busy admission ward, just getting a group to sit in the same room for half an hour can be a challenge. It is usually only after patients have shown some ability to work cooperatively with others in activity groups that the occupational therapist would propose cognitive behavioural group work as an appropriate treatment.

White and Freeman (2000) and Jones et al. (2000) among others demonstrated cognitive behavioural therapy to be effective in helping many clients overcome a wide range of problems. Forensic patients, by definition, have exhibited behaviours inconsistent with acceptable societal norms and are consequently stigmatized and isolated from society. Their adaptive engagement in occupational behaviours is dependent upon their recognition of the need to change, hence the critical need to engage clients actively in the process of change.

This chapter will briefly explore the theoretical underpinnings of cognitive behavioural therapy and the specific advantages of employing group therapy as an effective treatment medium with forensic patients. The interested reader is encouraged to explore in more depth some of the techniques commonly used with different problems.

Theory

The application of Beck's (1976) cognitive model is fundamental to a cognitive behavioural approach to treatment. The cognitive model postulates a link between the cognitive appraisal or thoughts (Lazarus 1991) one has about an event or a situation (the trigger), the feelings that are generated because of those thoughts and the behaviour that is exhibited as a result of these interactions. Behaviour will be based on what the individual considers will achieve the best result. Consequences occur as a result of any behaviour, and long-term consequences will often be ignored to allow the individual to receive immediate gratification. These aspects of the cognitive model can be viewed as a self-perpetuating cycle that needs to be broken to facilitate change.

Types of group programme

The types of cognitive behavioural treatment currently available at the Oxford Clinic are shown in Table 7.1. The list is not intended to be exhaustive but rather to offer a starting point for readers to explore the different techniques and have access to practical texts that offer guidance.

Table 7.1 Cognitive behavioural therapy interventions used in the Oxford Clinic for mentally disordered offenders

Intervention	Types of problem	Strategies	References
Anger control training	Poor impulse control Explosive anger Threatening non-verbal behaviour Projection of blame Lack of assertiveness Poor problem-solving skills	Anger diaries Consequential thinking/cost: benefit analysis Identification of faulty cognitions/self-calming statements High-risk situations Physiological arousal reduction Lifestyle change Role playing and video feedback Relapse prevention plan	Williams and Barlow (1998) Goldstein et al. (1998)

Table 7.1 (Contd)

Intervention	Types of problem	Strategies	References
Enhanced thinking skills	Offending behaviours Limited, narrow thinking styles Impulsive behaviour Poor problem-solving Lack of social skills Poor perspective taking	Creative thinking exercises Consequential thinking Problem-solving Goal setting Social skills training Moral reasoning Role shifts	Offending Behaviours Unit (2000) De Bono (1994)
Relapse prevention	Addictive behaviours	ABC of addictions Cravings diary Lifestyle change and goal setting Challenging cognitive distortions and justificatons Positive addictions Consequential thinking	Marlatt and Gordon (1985) Greanias and Seigel (2000)
Symptoms management	Active resistant psychotic symptoms Poor/erratic compliance	Education Physiological arousal reduction 'distraction' e.g. use of microphones Physical activity Indulgence Socialization Cognitive control Early warning signs Relapse prevention Problem-solving Social skills training	Chadwick et al. (1996) Kingdon and Turkington (1994)
Assertiveness training	Poor self-esteem Passivity/aggression Manipulation	Negotiation Compromise Personal rights Role play/video feedback Confidence building	Holland and Ward (2001)
Stress management	High levels of tension Chronic anxiety Poor problem-solving skills Avoidance behaviour	Physiological arousal reducton Goal setting Problem-solving Pleasurable activity Graded task assignments Self-calming statements	Whitehead and Adams (1996) Powell and Enright (1990)

Case example

Peter, a man in his late 30s, has a long history of alcohol abuse, plus a forensic history of burglary, assaults and car crime, and a diagnosis of late-onset paranoid schizophrenia with underlying antisocial personality disorder. At the time of his index offence he had become paranoid about a member of care staff whom he severely assaulted. Peter was initially very reluctant to acknowledge any problems that could not be blamed on others. His cognitive understanding of the problem was that the victim was responsible for not caring enough. His own drinking was not a problem as it was a normal activity for someone working in the building trade. His offending behaviour was reasonable because he only targeted banks or people who could afford the loss (and anyway the main problem was getting caught) and his mental illness was a stress reaction that did not require any treatment. On many occasions he has attempted or succeeded in absconding to obtain alcohol.

Peter has attended many cognitive behavioural therapy groups. These aimed to improve his anger control and problem-solving skills. He has also worked on individual relapse prevention strategies. Through these, he has begun to recognize some of his thoughts that resulted in his unhelpful and violent behaviours. He recognizes that his drinking is impulsive and related to ideas of entitlement ('I deserve a treat') and that his behaviour in hospital has had a direct effect on his lack of progress. On one occasion, he described working through his cognitive processes when feeling compelled to abscond. He challenged his beliefs that he was 'entitled to a holiday' and thought about the consequences in terms of his future and his desire to leave hospital. On this occasion it did not stop him giving in to his impulsiveness, but he returned the same day of his own accord and reflected on the whole episode, which was something he had never been able to do before.

Maladaptive characteristics

Types of common maladaptive characteristics that offending patients may possess also reflect those commonly seen in personality disorder, and include:

Impulsiveness There is often a strong tendency to jump to negative conclusions about a situation and react without thinking. Impulsive individuals have difficulty stopping to think and consequently have few problem-solving skills. They can experience difficulty in identifying their own thought processes. Engagement in high-risk behaviour results from a lack of judgement and poor problem-solving skills. One of the most important individual factors in offending is high impulsivity (Farrington 1996).

Case example

Jane, a female patient with borderline personality disorder, would consistently react to any hint of criticism or belief that she was being ignored by impulsively storming out of groups and refusing to attend activities, even those she enjoyed. She consequently found it difficult to manage her behaviour until she learnt, through group work, that she tended to avoid situations and inappropriately sought attention when experiencing emotional turmoil. This behaviour was not helpful for her self-confidence or her relationships with the other group members.

Lack of perspective taking Actions and reactions tend to be based on what feels right for the individual. Little account is taken of the impact of their behaviour on others. Often this is because of a genuine difficulty to see others' points of view or feelings (Chandler 1973). Moral reasoning training is a potential treatment to developing empathy skills and is a key part of the package delivered in the Aggression Replacement Training (Goldstein et al. 1998) and the Enhanced Thinking Skills programme (Offending Behaviours Programme Unit 2000). Using techniques such as role shifts has resulted in some patients either identifying with 'characters'' feelings from their own experiences or being surprised by understanding how another 'character' with whom they had little original allegiance might be feeling. One patient who had experienced terrible abuse in his past and consequently became violent and assaultive acknowledged that he was able to identify with a protector role, as this had always been something he had wished others had done for him.

Denial of responsibility and projection of blame Typically, patients blame others and, therefore, problems are often externalized. This behaviour is linked to the rigid maintenance of unhelpful schema (Young 1999). Placing the responsibility for things that go wrong on to others is one way of sustaining feelings of self-worth and entitlement. This can be seen again with Jane, who would blame staff for her self-harming and impulsive behaviour as she believed that they did not care about her and deliberately set out to sabotage her. Treatment has focused on enabling her to challenge some of her unhelpful beliefs and extreme thinking and enable her to talk about feelings of a lack of self-worth and experiences of being ignored and abused as a child.

Interpersonal problems Difficulties in interpersonal relationships are common. Many patients are capable of superficial social exchange but experience difficulties in close or intimate relationships. This may result in many of their existing relationships being unfulfilling and limiting, with unhealthy family dynamics. Poor social skills, including a tendency towards either over- or underassertiveness, poor conversational abilities, and difficulty establishing a range of alternative coping strategies are common problems for patients.

Rigidity Rigid thinking processes are particularly associated with personality disorder and are often seen within a medium secure service. Inflexible attitudes, beliefs and behaviours are difficult to change and are actively maintained. Creative thinking skills and the recognition and ability to challenge distorted cognition are essential to offer patients realistic possibilities for change.

The challenges of group work

There are many potential challenges in using cognitive behavioural therapy group work for occupational therapists.

Therapeutic use of self The relationship that the therapist develops with a group of clients has great potential to facilitate change. These skills are central to the role of the occupational therapist. The therapist needs to be self-aware and able to reflect. Use of teaching, role modelling and inductive facilitative skills, known as Socratic questioning (see Table 7.2), (Beck 1976) allows patients to explore and practise new skills and behaviours. The skills needed by the therapist are particularly important in a forensic setting where patients are detained against their will. This may affect their willingness to engage in therapeutic groups. Alternatively, drawing from personal experience, some clients may feel compelled to attend, not from internal motivation but from external expectations placed on them. This pressure to participate comes from the clinical team and the knowledge that engagement is the only route to discharge. Because of this, cognitive behavioural group work can be a very frustrating experience and therapists need to be realistic in their expectations for client change.

Because of the challenges and frustrations associated with their work, therapists should always have access to good supervisory networks for support and guidance.

Case example

Terry had successfully completed a relapse prevention programme and acknowledged the role that his drinking had played in his assaults on and eventual murder of his mother. He had made a commitment to avoid alcohol in the future, as he appeared to be aware of the risks alcohol presented to him and others. Some months later he was stating that he fully intended to drink on discharge and that drinking had never resulted in his becoming violent. Other group members effectively challenged him, but it became clear that treatment had had little impact on the likelihood of changing his future behaviour. It is always important to be aware that patients can 'learn' to give the expected responses, and therapists need to be realistic in their goals.

Cohesion Cohesiveness is one of the key goals of group therapy. The greater the degree of cohesion, the greater is the ability for the group to contain individual differences and prevent isolation (White and Freeman 2000). A cohesive group is one in which members share common goals and care about each other's progress and development. Typically, forensic patients have some difficulty recognizing the needs of others.

Task focus Cognitive behavioural therapy is a process by which clients identify problems and seek to find a resolution (White and Freeman 2000). In this way, goals are explicit and outcomes clear. Often patients have difficulty seeing beyond their goal of leaving the secure setting and achieving freedom. Working together towards a common goal presents its own challenges when many of the patients have never had the experience of effective teamwork. The skill of the therapist is balancing the need for cohesion with the importance of task focus to enable optimum group functioning.

Limitations of the environment Within medium security, there exists a strong containing element. The structures that are inherent in any institutional setting are heightened within secure environments. All aspects of existence are governed by the necessity to maintain safety, and patients have little opportunity to empower themselves. Consequences of relapse are serious and the process of risk assessment and management means that access to most of the opportunities we take for granted are not available to this group. Engagement in treatment is considered by the clinical team to be critical. This often results in attendance at groups because of external control. It is the therapist's responsibility to attempt to empower patients and enable them to own their problems before they can actively engage. Often patients do not view the occupational therapist as an authority figure in the same way that they view the doctors and nurses. It has often been said to me that the occupational therapists are 'different' from other members of the team. Patients tend to view occupational therapists differently because we are associated with offering time and pleasurable activity. This can be an advantage in engaging the patient in treatment.

In addition to the problems of engagement, a secure environment cannot be considered as a fair reflection of society. To a large extent, we learn to adapt to our environment. Patients have expressed a reluctance to show any negative emotional content such as anger or frustration for fear of being negatively evaluated by staff. They often believe that the consequences of expressing feelings will be punishment through loss of leave, status, or delay in discharge. This can result in 'model' behaviour that is not representative of their real life in the community. Terry demonstrated this by presenting a reassuring picture of a man who had made good progress in understanding his problems while on the ward but quickly reverted to alcohol when given the first opportunity when on leave. Cognitive behavioural group work is based on problem identification and resolution; it requires patients to develop a new skill base and to practise changing cognitive appraisal and adaptive behaviours.

Planning a group

Whatever the type of group, to ensure it will be as effective as possible, the therapist must take into consideration a number of issues.

Facilitators It is always recommended that two people run the programme and they should both have knowledge and experience of cognitive behavioural techniques. This enables the sharing of facilitative roles and responsibilities, helps with feedback and reflection and the planning required after a session. I have found that this patient group can be enormously challenging. Working with another experienced colleague helps maintain therapist focus and motivation. In the Oxford Clinic we work closely with the clinical psychology department and will usually aim to have at least one member from each discipline facilitating. This broadens and enriches the group experience as each discipline brings different perspectives and skills to bear. This can have many benefits, as the occupational therapist can be very effective at motivating attendees, coordinating and running the group and addressing environmental considerations, while the psychologist can offer specific expertise in assessment and psychological evaluation. Providing training places in groups for professionals to develop their skills has proved to be an invaluable way of both increasing knowledge and application within the larger staff group and providing continuity in treatment when one of the lead therapists is not available.

Duration of treatment Usually, cognitive behavioural programmes are time limited, lasting between eight and 20 sessions. This is dependent on the focus of the group and the capacity of the group members. Each session can last from 45 minutes to one and a half hours. It is important that the group discusses any changes to the schedule that was initially agreed. In my experience, being clear about how many sessions will be offered can be the deciding factor in whether a patient agrees to attend.

One salutary lesson was learned when the service was offering a number of cognitive behavioural treatments at the same time. We found that patients had no difficulty processing information from one group, but when they were attending several they described feeling confused and demoralized. One patient asked which group he was in and could not remember what he was supposed to be discussing. We now try to help patients focus on one identified problem at a time and build on their knowledge with subsequent courses.

Patient selection Consideration must be given to the number, homogeneity, nature and degree of disorder, as well as the cognitive capacity, of the group. Five to ten group members constitute an acceptable number. Too few patients will limit the potential for growth, and too many can weaken its ability to focus on a task. The presence of active mental illness or severe personality disorder increases the potential for dropout. The degree to which patients share similar characteristics must be considered. Issues such as the risk of reinforcing negative behaviours can be a problem unless managed well by the therapist. Patients who self-harm can become competitive and accuse one another of attention-seeking behaviour. Nevertheless, it is important that patients can identify shared experience and have some capacity to consider others for the group to develop any cohesion.

The gender mix and nature of past offending behaviours are also important. Most of the women with whom I have worked have not expressed concern about working with men in the same group, unless the men have perpetrated sexual abuse. This is usually because of the woman's own experiences of abuse and victimization. Nevertheless, we do seek to provide specific group programmes for women, although there are often too few to make a large enough group.

Most patients have little choice but to live together within the same unit. This inevitably causes some problems in encouraging honest disclosure. Patients are often either very critical or judgemental of each other, or have a tendency to minimize or project blame. Exploring prejudice and the dangers of minimizing their own behaviour is important for patients to acknowledge the need for change.

The degree to which a patient is unable to engage fully due to the active presence of mental illness or disorder must be considered when designing a programme. Acute illness greatly influences an individual's capacity to organize or control cognitive capacity, hence learning is inhibited. I have found the patients most appropriate for cognitive behavioural group work are those whose illness or disorder is stabilized. A group can contain a small number of patients with residual symptoms, but active illness inhibits the group's ability to focus on tasks.

Group venues There may be difficulties in finding a suitable venue in which to run a group. Consideration must be given to ensure that therapists and patients are safe and that other colleagues are aware of the location. Security is in part guided by the development of a safe psychological environment for the individual, where they feel contained by the therapist. Space is always at a premium, but it is essential that there is enough room for active role playing, a core strategy for learning adaptive techniques.

Assessment and evaluation Before and after cognitive behavioural programmes, the therapist needs to consider assessment procedures. These can include pre- and post-group psychometric questionnaires relating to the particular issue being addressed by the group. In the Oxford Clinic, the psychology team coordinates these assessments. In addition to these assessments, patients are asked to consider developing their own objectives and are regularly asked for feedback on the usefulness of the group content. This allows the therapist to evaluate the programme and incorporate the feedback into future groups.

Throughout the course of the group, a series of homework tasks are given to the patients. This enables therapists and other group members to monitor progress and motivation in the intervening time between groups. Experience indicates many patients will 'forget' to address these, and this is usually a good indicator as to their level of engagement. At the end of a time-limited group, patients will be asked to evaluate learning, and therapists will prepare a report on each individual's progress based on the formal assessments, therapist's impressions, the patient's personal evaluations and achievement of objectives. This process is an open one, and reports are available to the patient to comment on.

Motivation There is simply no better way to engage the patient than to sit down and explore their personal needs openly and honestly with them on an individual basis. All treatment should reflect the aims of the individual, and the first stage involves problem recognition. This can be a difficult process with some of the patients who fail to recognize having problems they need to address. In these cases, the therapist is challenged with helping the individual to identify intrinsic and extrinsic motivators (Oliver 1993). Intrinsically, this may be by arousing the patient's interest and curiosity and beliefs that change is in their best interest and, extrinsic-ally, that active participation will improve their chances of discharge or other positive incentives will be available. A degree of choice is essential to an effective group, and there is little point forcing a patient to attend.

Once the patient has engaged, the skill of the therapist and the experi-ence of being part of a meaningful group will hopefully engage the patient further. A particularly effective means by which we encourage per-sonal motivation and active involvement is through a process of inclusion. We attempt to encourage all staff and patients to view inclusion in the groups as a positive step that reflects the progress of the individual. We provide all potential group members and key team members such as pri-mary nurses and medical staff with written information. If everyone believes the group to have significant value, it will be treated with respect. Personal experience suggests those who engage will share with others their learning experiences and help generalize some of the techniques on a day-to-day basis within the ward. Patients can be heard discussing the group with others and suggesting that they might benefit from some of the techniques. Peer pressure and competitiveness have a strong role to play, and the therapist can direct this positively, for example to improve attendance and the completion of homework exercises.

Socratic questioning Of all the techniques I have used with an offending patient group, Socratic inquiry has been the most useful (Beck 1976). Its aim is to facilitate learning and disclosure using systematic questioning and inductive reasoning. It is particularly helpful in avoiding conflict in general interpersonal relationships and encourages the patient to devel-op independent thinking skills and separate facts from beliefs and opinions. Patients often actively challenge the therapist and hold on rigid-ly to their belief systems. Socratic questioning encourages them to consider some of their unhelpful beliefs and attitudes. Socratic question-ing consists of certain types of open-ended questions identified in Table 7.2, which gives explanations and examples.

Table 7.2 Socratic questioning (adapted from Beck 1976)

Type of question	Explanation	Example
Memory	Recall of information (including thoughts and feelings)	'What did you do when he said that?' 'What were you thinking?'
Translation	Changing information or ideas to ensure proper understanding	'How can you relate this with that?'

Table 7.2 (Contd)

Type of question	Explanation	Example
Interpretation	To discover the relationship between facts, generalizations, values and beliefs	'In what way do you think that that behaviour is similar to your offending behaviour?' 'Where else in your life have you felt like this?'
Application	Application of skills to a specific situation or problem	'What else could you do to change it?' 'What did you learn from that?'
Analysis	Problem-solving and objectivity Reasoning skills	'What do you think is causing this problem and how do you know whether you are right or wrong?' 'What evidence do you have that this is true?'
Synthesis	Creative thinking	'How else could you think about the situation?' 'What other reasons might be had for doing that?'
Evaluation	Value judgements based on personal standards Clarifying thoughts and feelings	'What do you look for in a friendship and why?'

Conclusion

Cognitive behavioural group work with forensic patients is a very challenging intervention. It is often frustrating and demoralizing, and changes are small and slow. Nevertheless, with a good, committed team of therapy staff it can offer great rewards when patients do reflect on themselves and their behaviour. For example, Tony, a patient who has actively engaged in treatment, has consistently stated how much he has changed, and this is borne out in his general behaviour and use of positive coping mechanisms while in hospital. His assertiveness skills have improved, and he is now able to access his thinking and demonstrate the ability to problem solve on his own. His levels of impulsiveness have reduced, and he is able to seek help when he feels under too much pressure. The challenge for him is to learn to generalize this into other environments when he leaves hospital.

It may be suggested by some that occupational therapists may not be adequately trained in offering cognitive behavioural treatments. Their professional education does incorporate training on cognitive approaches and client-centred techniques that are well suited to a cognitive behavioural approach. There are also opportunities to extend these skills through postgraduate education. Also, there is no substitute for experiential learning with good supervision by experienced staff. The particular skills that the occupational therapist has with regard to group work and the use of activity to facilitate change makes them ideally suited to run cognitive behavioural group programmes.

This chapter has aimed to help the occupational therapist develop an understanding of some of the complex problems of the forensic patient and consider some of the therapeutic issues of setting up a cognitive behavioural group work programme in a secure environment. It is hoped that the use of examples from the practice setting reflects both the frustrations and the rewards of working with the mentally disordered offender and offers the reader some tools with which to enhance their practice.

References

Beck A (1976) Cognitive Therapy and the Emotional Disorders. New York: International Universities Press.

Chadwick P, Birchwood M and Trower P (1996) Cognitive Therapy for Delusions, Voices and Paranoia. Chichester: John Wiley.

Chandler MJ (1973) Egocentrism and antisocial behaviour: The assessment and training of social perspective-taking skills. Developmental Psychology (9) 326–332.

De Bono E (1994) De Bono's Thinking Course. London: BBC Consumer Publishing (books).

Farrington D (1996) Criminal Psychology: Individual and family factors in the explanation and prevention of offending. In: Working with Offenders: Psychological Practice in Offender Rehabilitation, Hollin C (ed.). Chichester: John Wiley.

Goldstein A, Glick B and Gibbs J (1998) Aggression Replacement Training. Illinois: Research Press.

Greanias T and Seigal S (2000) 'Dual Diagnosis'. In: Cognitive-Behavioural Group Therapy for Specific Problems and Populations, White J and Freeman A (eds.). Washington DC: American Psychological Association.

Holland S and Ward C (2001) Assertiveness: A Practical Approach. Bicester: Speechmark.

Jones C, Cormac I, Mota J and Campbell C (2000) Cognitive Behaviour Therapy for Schizophrenia (Cochrane Review). The Cochrane Library, Issue 4 Oxford: Update Software.

Kingdon D and Turkington D (1994) Cognitive Behavioural Therapy of Schizophrenia. Hove: Psychology Press.

Lazarus R (1991) Cognition and motivation in emotion. American Psychologist 46(4) 352–367.

CHAPTER 8

Evaluation of forensic occupational therapy practice

CHANNINE CLARKE

Introduction

In the current health and social care climate, where health professionals are increasingly being asked to demonstrate their value and effectiveness, evaluation of service provision is essential for occupational therapists. It is more than the appraisal of clinical effectiveness. Evaluation of services enables therapists to examine not only changes that have occurred for clients, themselves and the service but also what led to those changes. Through the use of tools such as outcome measurement, clinical audit, involvement of service users and evidence-based practice, therapists are able to evaluate their services, improve the quality of care for their clients and demonstrate clinical effectiveness to service users, carers, managers, commissioners and the general public. This chapter aims to discuss the ways in which therapists can evaluate the quality and effectiveness of occupational therapy services within forensic psychiatry.

Measuring outcomes

In order to provide evidence about the clinical effectiveness of occupational therapy, practitioners should be evaluating the outcomes of their intervention. Outcomes are the final result, or consequences, of intervention and can be defined as 'changes in a person's status that can confidently be attributed to the preceding intervention/s' (College of Occupational Therapists 2001 p.5). For occupational therapists, this means that they should be assessing meaningful changes (outcomes) that have taken place for their clients as a result of occupational therapy intervention.

With the current emphasis on high quality service provision, occupational therapists can use outcome measurement as a way of ensuring that they are providing an effective, efficient and appropriate service for their forensic clients. Through outcome measurement, therapists are able to:

- evaluate the effects of occupational therapy service provision
- demonstrate progress to clients
- modify intervention programmes to be meaningful to service users
- eliminate wasteful or ineffective intervention strategies
- plan future service developments
- predict the effects of intervention for future service users
- provide evidence to support practice.

Within forensic psychiatry, there are various outcomes that a client or therapist may expect. Examples include: increased independence in activities of daily living, improved social skills, decreased anger or anxiety, decreased level of security or perceived risk, improved mental health status, attainment of treatment goals/objectives, improved satisfaction with the service or better quality of life and community discharge.

One of the difficulties that therapists face when measuring outcomes is the uncertainty about whether or not it is occupational therapy intervention that has brought about a change in a client's status. This is a problem that all professionals encounter and is not unique to occupational therapists. For example, while other team members may believe that it is medication, psychological intervention, counselling or the passage of time that has brought about change in a client, therapists could argue that it has been brought about by occupational therapy. However, unless only one intervention has been provided, the reality in practice is that a patient's progress is likely to be a combination of the various treatments and therapies available to them. It is therefore very difficult for any one professional to state that their intervention has brought about such progress. While occupational therapists should, where possible, continue to utilize outcome measures in order to help them provide evidence regarding their clinical effectiveness, there may also be a need to consider working collaboratively with other professionals to measure the outcomes of the multidisciplinary team.

This can be demonstrated by an example drawn from personal experience of working in a small rehabilitation hostel. There a team of four multidisciplinary staff measures the outcomes of care for the patients. Patients' goals are reviewed each month. Some aspects of care can be measured with regards to the effectiveness of occupational therapy, for example the ability of a patient to cook independently, following six individual sessions. However, it is the view of the staff at the hostel that, as long as the patient achieves the specified team goals, it is not necessary to be so specific about which professional facilitated that achievement.

Feedback from hostel residents is that for them it is 'getting better' and reaching their goals that is important, not which one of the staff enabled them to do that.

Outcome measures tend to fall into four main categories (College of Occupational Therapists 2001), namely those that measure:

Changes in function, health or quality of life – these evaluate changes in a client's physical, psychological or social well-being or quality of life. Therapists would need to ensure that they had established a baseline assessment prior to intervention in order to compare levels of function, mental health status, etc. before and after occupational therapy intervention. Such measures may also be used to help therapists compare the effectiveness of different interventions, that is comparing outcomes of clients who received different interventions or comparing outcomes with those who did not receive intervention. Therapists using these types of measure need to be aware that the reliability of the results may be affected if evaluating an individual whose mental health status fluctuates daily. 'Before and after' measures may not therefore be the most appropriate type to use in acute forensic settings but could be used in conjunction with other measures like goal attainment to provide more accurate measures of outcome.

Goal attainment – these measure the extent to which a client's goals were achieved through occupational therapy intervention. For example, goal attainment would involve measuring whether, following occupational therapy, a client was able to 'independently cook their evening meal' or 'engage in a social board game for an hour with three other people'. When evaluating goal attainment, it is important that therapists make sure that achievement of the goals has had an 'occupational impact' on the client, that is, is the client now able to carry out daily living tasks which they were previously unable to perform (College of Occupational Therapists 2001)?

Client satisfaction – measures the level of client/carer satisfaction with the intervention or service received. In order to use satisfaction as a measure of how successful occupational therapy intervention has been, it is important that therapists ask the client/carer whether the intervention or care received means that they are now able to perform tasks that they couldn't before. It is only by asking such questions that relate to outcomes of intervention that therapists will be able to evaluate the effectiveness of intervention and service provision.

Population changes in health-related areas – these are more general measures, which provide information about service outcomes for groups of clients. For example, measuring outcomes such as number of referrals and re-referrals, discharges and placements, lengths of time in occupational therapy, relapses or suicide rates may assist therapists planning future service provision. Again, this area also lends itself to multidisciplinary evaluation as many of these changes are within limited control of the occupational therapist and affect the whole team.

There are a number of standardized assessments and outcome measures available to occupational therapists working in forensic psychiatry, although the majority are not specific to the field or to occupational therapy. In order to select the right outcome measure, therapists need to be clear about what and whose outcomes they want to measure, that is client, therapist, group, multidisciplinary team or service, level of function, goal attainment or satisfaction, etc. Once this is decided, a review of the various measures will enable therapists to ascertain whether particular measures will provide the required information. A comprehensive guide to outcome measurement, which includes a list of measures commonly used by forensic occupational therapists, is published by the College of Occupational Therapists (2001).

Clinical audit

Clinical audit can be used by forensic occupational therapists to systematically evaluate the quality of care that they provide for clients. It is defined by the Department of Health (1993, cited in College of Occupational Therapists 1998a p.1) as 'the systematic and critical analysis of the quality of clinical care including diagnostic and treatment procedures, associated use of resources, outcomes and quality of life for clients'. This 'analysis' involves comparing practice against pre-defined standards to ensure that they are being achieved and that quality services are being maintained.

With Government (Department of Health 1998a, 2000a, 2000b) putting quality high on the agenda, clinical audit provides an important tool for evaluating the quality of clinical care, monitoring attainment of standards and subsequently improving the quality of our professional practice. As it is the responsibility of all occupational therapists to ensure that they are providing a high quality service for their clients, clinical audit has an essential role to play in evaluating and improving practice within the field of forensic psychiatry. Many aspects of forensic occupational therapy service provision can be evaluated. Examples from practice at the hostel include auditing:

• **evidence of the use of models of practice**, e.g. literature to support the use of models, documentation regarding the application of models to the client group, evidence that assessments are underpinned by a model of practice.

- **use of assessments,** e.g. auditing the ability of staff to demonstrate their clinical reasoning for their choice of assessments, participation of occupational therapy staff in multidisciplinary risk assessment, that local criteria for assessment has been adhered to, assessment findings are recorded and there is evidence of re-evaluation.
- **documentation,** e.g. staff adhere to College of Occupational Therapists' core standards on record keeping
- **intervention,** e.g. measurable goals are identified based on assessment findings, there is evidence of a patient's involvement in treatment planning and there are written protocols for each therapeutic activity provided
- **evaluation,** e.g. there is evidence of the use of outcome measures, patient involvement in evaluating their therapy is documented, discharge summaries are provided, regular forums for service evaluation take place with patients and staff, there is ongoing clinical audit activity
- **staff competence,** e.g. all staff are able to demonstrate evidence of continuing professional development, there are records of regular staff training.

Such audits have enabled therapists not only to identify areas for improvement but also to demonstrate how effective and efficient services are and highlight current areas of good practice. This has had a positive impact on clients where benefits such as improved assessment procedures, more appropriate referrals, use of the most effective interventions, better information for clients, more consistent teamwork and increased competence all lead to a higher quality of service for clients.

Although the emphasis of clinical audit is on evaluation of clinical care, practitioners can audit various aspects of forensic occupational therapy services. Donabedian (1964) in College of Occupational Therapists (1998a) provides a useful framework for therapists at the hostel through which they have been able to reflect on service evaluation, namely structure, process and outcome.

Structure: this has involved evaluating/auditing organizational factors such as resources, environment and safety, for example auditing security procedures, staffing levels, skill mix, use of control and restraint and seclusion, violence and aggression, available resources and use of clinical areas.

Process: includes treatment delivery, interactions between staff and clients and access to services. Process audits have included evaluating referrals, assessment procedures, clinical interventions and treatment techniques, documentation, the care programme approach, caseloads, communication with the multidisciplinary team and user involvement with their care.

Outcomes: this has enabled therapists to evaluate changes in a client's status as a result of preceding occupational therapy intervention, for example goal achievement, discharge, patient compliance, re-admission rates and client satisfaction with groups, and individual therapies.

The College of Occupational Therapists' (2002) *Standards of Practice for Occupational Therapists Working in Forensic Residential Settings* should be used to guide practice and facilitate the audit of forensic services. Other national standards such as the *National Service Framework for Mental Health* (Department of Health 1998b) should also be integral to practice and audited to ensure that therapists are adhering to the national agenda.

To guide practitioners through the process of audit and ensure that audits at the hostel bring about desired improvements in the care of patients, the occupational therapists familiarized themselves with the 'audit cycle'. This is exemplified through an audit carried out at the hostel.

1. Selecting an appropriate topic – it was decided to audit whether patients were being involved in decisions regarding their therapy at the hostel. This topic was chosen as a result of concerns raised by patients that they were not always been included in these decisions. This audit received priority as the College of Occupational Therapists' (2000) *Code of Ethics and Professional Conduct* clearly identifies the need for collaborative practice between therapists and patients when planning therapy.
2. Deciding who should be involved – an audit group was set up that included hostel staff, the hostel manager and the patients (the hostel has four patients).
3. Setting standards – measurable standards of practice were negotiated and agreed upon by the audit group and clearly documented.
4. Choosing methods of data collection – it was agreed that occupational therapy records would be reviewed for evidence of patient involvement in planning their therapy, and patients would be asked whether they had been involved in such decisions.
5. Collecting the data – two staff and two patients were chosen by the audit group to collect the data over a period of one month.
6. Analysis of data – data were returned to the audit group for analysis.
7. Identifying changes and required action – points for action emerged from the data. For example, writing the treatment goals from the perspective of the patient and not the treatment goals of the therapists, the

need for the signature of the patient on the treatment plan, the need for a regular review of this process.

8. Implementing changes – changes were implemented over the following six months.
9. Re-auditing to evaluate whether changes have made a difference – a re-audit took place six months later to see whether the implemented changes had brought about the desired change. It was agreed that regular audit would take place annually.

A useful resource is the College of Occupational Therapists' (1998a) *Clinical Audit Information Pack*. This provides an easy-to-use, step-by-step guide to planning and carrying out a clinical audit. It includes a ten-point checklist outlining factors that need to be considered in order to successfully complete each stage of the audit cycle.

Within forensic psychiatry, occupational therapists work with a client group that has complex and diverse needs. Individual service users' mental health status may fluctuate on a daily basis. Additionally, environmental influences, such as levels of security, have a significant impact on a client's behaviour, mental state and level of function. All these issues need to be considered when planning an audit in a forensic unit in order to identify what should be audited and how relevant and useful information can be collected in a constantly changing environment. While this may appear to be challenging, it is a task that therapists need to accept. Otherwise there is a danger that therapists will audit only aspects of a service that are unaffected by such issues, and not focus on trying to evaluate the process and outcomes of therapeutic intervention.

User involvement in evaluation

Central to high quality healthcare is service user involvement. With the Government's commitment to developing services that are sensitive and responsive to the needs of patients, occupational therapists should be ensuring that patients are engaged in planning, implementing and evaluating their care. Forensic patients have a fundamental right to be involved in decisions that affect their lives. With their own expertise about how their mental disorder affects their function, they can make significant contributions to planning and evaluating their therapy, of which they have first-hand experience.

Literature has highlighted how user involvement increases clinical effectiveness. Advantages include: improved communication between staff and patient, increased staff awareness of the patients' 'illness experience', greater patient compliance with treatment, increased patient satisfaction with service provision, increased feelings of empowerment, autonomy, confidence and control, and a more responsive, cost-effective service (Department of Health 1999a, National Schizophrenia Fellowship 1997, Took 1999). Such benefits subsequently lead to improved health outcomes and a greater quality of life for the patient.

For forensic patients, involvement in decision-making processes and service evaluation has often been avoided due to doubts about the patient's credibility as a result of illness, appearance and hospitalization (Woodside 1991). Furthermore, models of practice within forensic institutions have historically been medically orientated with a paternalistic approach to treatment, prescription of care and an expectation of patient compliance (Charles et al. 1999, Kee 1996). Subsequently, patients have little experience of being active partners in decisions regarding their treatment and become passive recipients of treatment. This is a particular issue for forensic patients who have been detained in a secure environment, usually against their will and had many decisions taken away from them. Musker and Bryne (1997) highlight how custodial care creates an imbalance of power relations between patient and staff. Simple decisions, such as being able to go to the bathroom alone, going out for a walk, choosing when to eat, have been taken away. This results in feelings of disempowerment. The lack of patient involvement in decisions regarding their treatment and care throughout their stay in hospital can only exacerbate this, leading to feelings of helplessness, hopelessness, disempowerment and deterioration in their mental health.

All forensic healthcare professionals, including occupational therapists, need to examine their own values and behaviours regarding user involvement. Many may feel discomfort and professionally threatened or disempowered by engaging the patient as an active partner (Law et al. 1995, Kent and Read 1998). Within forensic psychiatry, staff need to reflect on their attitudes towards patients who have a history of violence and offending behaviour. Otherwise, potentially negative feelings such as fear, revulsion or anxiety can lead to further exclusion of the patient from involvement in their care (Kumar 2000). Supervision plays an important part in allowing occupational therapy staff to reflect on and monitor such issues (College of Occupational Therapists 1997).

There is a balance to be made between user involvement and security. This can lead to a conflict where occupational therapists are willing to involve the patient in decisions about their care but are constrained perhaps by the environment, policies, procedures or legislation. For example, the client may believe themselves ready to have greater access to the nearby town and discuss the appropriateness of this at their stage of rehabilitation with the occupational therapist. Despite their agreement, the Home Office may not sanction this. While occupational therapy's code of ethics encourages user involvement and collaborative practice, there is also a responsibility to the safety of the community. One unpublished study (Clarke 2002) identifies a split between the patient's expressed desire for increased involvement in decisions about their care and the majority of the staff's belief that such an increase is not viable. This they attribute to the constraints of legislation, the fact that the patients have committed an offence and the potential risks that they pose. The *Fallon Report* (Department of Health 1999b) criticized strategies for patient empowerment for people with severe personality disorder where insufficient checks were in place to ensure security. Such issues need further exploration to highlight the advantages and limitations to user involvement.

Occupational therapists, with their focus on empowerment and promotion of health and well-being, are ideally placed to help shift the culture of forensic institutions from paternalistic models towards a shared approach. It is important to provide opportunities for decision-making and to empower patients to direct their care and enable them to regain a sense of control over their lives. However, such a shift is likely to be slow as traditional practices are entrenched in current legislation and regulation. Nevertheless, involvement in care planning, case conferences, community meetings, activity planning meetings, forums, receiving copies of therapy plans, etc. are all ways in which such empowerment can be facilitated and users can have a say in evaluating practice.

It is acknowledged, however, that not all patients will want to be involved in all decisions regarding their therapy, for example those that feel too unwell or do not want the responsibility. In such cases, occupational therapists should ascertain how much involvement the patient wishes to have in their therapy, treatment plans and goals and keep them informed of decisions that have been made on their behalf. Brody (1980) highlights how failure to ascertain a patient's desire for involvement may have a significant effect on the therapeutic success of intervention. Occupational therapists also have a role to play in assisting patients to develop the skills necessary for effective involvement, for example in communication, negotiation and decision-making skills.

In addition to involvement in planning and evaluating therapy, occupational therapists should involve patients in evaluating service provision (Duff et al. 1996). Patients often provide different views of problems and offer new and innovative solutions (Department of Health 1999a) and as such should be active participants in the entire process. Reviewing patient satisfaction with services (Cleary 1999), involving patients in clinical audit (Kelson 1996, Avis 1997), research (Couldrick 2000), clinical guidelines (Duff et al. 1996) and evaluating therapeutic interventions enables therapists to assess whether they have provided a responsive and appropriate service.

Evidence-based practice

Evidence based practice plays an important part in evaluating forensic occupational therapy services. As they become more accountable for their services, practice must be underpinned by sound evidence so that therapists can confidently demonstrate that interventions being provided are correct and worthwhile (Taylor 1997, Bannigan 1997, Roberts and Barber 2001). This is reinforced in the profession's code of ethics (College of Occupational Therapists 2000 p.13), which states the responsibility of therapists to ensure that practice is 'evidence-based and consistent with research findings'. Therapists should therefore access literature, systematic reviews and research on a regular basis and integrate it into practice where appropriate. However, at present, there have been few studies on the effectiveness of forensic occupational therapy, but the evidence base is growing (College of Occupational Therapists 1998b). Forensic occupational therapists must engage in and disseminate research in order to provide future evidence.

Therapists also have an individual responsibility, as part of their continuing professional development, to keep up to date with practice, undertake ongoing learning, and take time to reflect on practice (College of Occupational Therapists 2000). To facilitate service evaluation, therapists need to familiarize themselves with information technology. Such resources as the Internet and literature databases enable therapists to evaluate the effectiveness of interventions, see what other forensic therapists are providing, and seek up-to-date information on therapies.

While strong emphasis is placed on the effectiveness and efficiency of service provision there are only limited resources, and therapists need to consider how this may affect practice. Increasingly, therapists may experience a conflict between what is expected from them in practice (from managers and commissioners) and their core values and beliefs. Within forensic units, the holistic approach adopted by therapists is often in contrast to the medical model adopted by the medical and nursing teams. Therapists have to consider how they can provide an effective and efficient service when those purchasing the service have medically orientated priorities and deploy resources to facilitate medical intervention and early discharge. This may leave few resources to address occupational and social needs. Therapists therefore have to decide which interventions will be provided first, leading to a possible conflict between patient expectations and inadequate resources (Pringle 1996). To address this, therapists need to be stating the purpose and objectives of their service and engaging in the activities outlined here to ensure their service is appropriate to the needs of the patient population.

Conclusion

In summary, it is clear that occupational therapists must now be evaluating their practice and service provision to ensure clinical effectiveness. As forensic occupational therapists, we have a responsibility to patients to make sure that the therapy we offer is as effective as possible and that their opinions and choices are integrated into treatment and service planning in order to provide a responsive, needs-led service. This is not something that should be left to occupational therapy managers but is the responsibility of all therapy staff and should be an integral part of their practice.

References

Avis M (1997) Incorporating patients' voices in the audit process. Quality in Health Care 6, 86–91.

Bannigan K (1997) Clinical effectiveness: Systematic reviews and evidence-based practice in occupational therapy. British Journal of Occupational Therapy 60 (11) 479–483.

Brody D (1980) The patients' role in clinical decision-making. Annals of Internal Medicine 93, 718–722.

Charles C, Whelan T and Gafni A (1999) What do we mean by partnership in making decisions about treatment? British Medical Journal 319: 780–782.

Clarke C (2002) Current and Desired Involvement of Forensic Mental Health Service Users in Decisions Regarding their Care. (COT Thesis Collection).

Cleary PD (1999) The increasing importance of patient surveys. Quality in Health Care 8, 212.

College of Occupational Therapists (1997) Statement on Supervision in Occupational Therapy. (SPP 150A). London: College of Occupational Therapists.

College of Occupational Therapists (1998a) Clinical Audit Information Pack. London: College of Occupational Therapists.

College of Occupational Therapists (1998b) Evidence-based Bulletin: Occupational Therapy in Forensic Settings. London: College of Occupational Therapists.

College of Occupational Therapists (1999) Clinical Governance: A Position Statement. London: College of Occupational Therapists.

College of Occupational Therapists (2000) Code of Ethics and Professional Conduct for Occupational Therapists. London: College of Occupational Therapists.

College of Occupational Therapists (2001) Outcome Measures Information Pack for Occupational Therapy. London: College of Occupational Therapists.

College of Occupational Therapists (2002) Standards of Practice for Occupational Therapists Working in Forensic Residential Settings. London: College of Occupational Therapists.

Couldrick L (2000) Consumer involvement in research: reflections of a professional. British Journal of Therapy and Rehabilitation 7 (7) 294–302.

Department of Health (1993) Clinical Audit: Meeting and Improving Standards in Healthcare. London: HMSO.

Department of Health (1998a) A First-class Service: Quality in the new NHS. London: HMSO.

Department of Health (1998b) National Service Framework for Mental Health. London: HMSO.

Department of Health (1999a) Patient and Public Involvement in the NHS. London: HMSO.

Department of Health (1999b) Executive Summary of the Report of the Committee of Inquiry into the Personality Disorder Unit, Ashworth Special Hospital, chaired by Peter Fallon QC. London: The Stationery Office.

Department of Health (2000a) A Quality Strategy for Social Care. London: HMSO.

Department of Health (2000b) The NHS Plan. London: HMSO.

Duff L, Kelson M, Marriott S, McIntosh A, Brown S, Cape J, Marcus N and Traynor M (1996) Clinical guidelines: involving patients and users of services. Journal of Clinical Effectiveness 1(3) 104–112.

Kee F (1996) Patient's prerogatives and perceptions of benefit. British Medical Journal 312: 958–960.

Kelson M (1996) User involvement in clinical audit: a review of developments and issues of good practice. Journal of Evaluation in Clinical Practice 2(2) 97–109.

Kent H and Read J (1998) Measuring consumer participation in mental health services: Are attitudes related to professional orientation? International Journal of Social Psychiatry 44(4) 295–310.

Kumar S (2000) Client empowerment in psychiatry and the professional abuse of clients: where do we stand? International Journal of Psychiatry in Medicine 30(1) 61–70.

Law M, Baptiste S and Mills J (1995) Client-centred practice: What does it mean and does it make a difference? Canadian Journal of Occupational Therapy 62(5) 250–257.

Musker M and Bryne M (1997) Applying empowerment in mental health practice. Nursing Standard 11(3) 45–47.

National Schizophrenia Fellowship (1997) How to Involve Service Users and Carers in Planning, Running and Monitoring Care Services and Curriculum Development. Surrey: National Schizophrenia Fellowship.

Pringle E (1996) Occupational therapy in the reformed NHS: The views of Therapists and Therapy Managers. British Journal of Occupational Therapy 59(9) 401–406.

Roberts A and Barber G (2001) Applying research evidence to practice. British Journal of Occupational Therapy 64(5) 223–227.

Taylor M (1997) What is evidence-based practice? British Journal of Occupational Therapy 69(11) 470–474.

Took M (1999) Involving service users and carers. Journal of Psychiatric and Mental Health Nursing (6) 485–487.

Woodside H (1991) The participation of mental health consumers in health care issues. Canadian Journal of Occupational Therapy 58(1) 3–5.

PART THREE

FORENSIC OCCUPATIONAL THERAPY IN OTHER SETTINGS

CHAPTER 9

Occupational therapy in a high-security hospital – the Broadmoor perspective

MICHELLE WALSH AND JOE AYRES

Introduction

In 1800, James Hadfield fired a pistol at King George III as he entered the royal box at the Theatre Royal Drury Lane. Following his 'not guilty' verdict 'by reason of insanity', there developed an awareness of the need to provide care for mentally disordered offenders. Broadmoor's origins stem from the Criminal Lunatic Asylums Act (1860), which made legal arrangements for the care of the criminally insane that had grown in number since their recognition in 1800. Broadmoor was founded in 1863, followed by Rampton Hospital, its northern equivalent in 1912 and Moss Side (now known as Ashworth Hospital) in 1914.

The 1959 Mental Health Act (revised in 1983) named the three institutions 'Special Hospitals' and defined their purpose. This was to provide for: 'persons subject to detention under the Mental Health Act (1959) who require treatment under conditions of special security on account of their dangerous, violent or criminal propensities'.

Broadmoor Hospital

Broadmoor Hospital provides specialist mental health care and treatment for men and women with an enduring mental illness and/or personality disorder whose individual needs require their care to be provided within a high-security environment. The hospital aims to provide a full range of treatments and therapeutic activities for patients including pre-admission advice to other agencies, comprehensive assessment of patients' mental illness and dangerousness, specialist treatment, care and rehabilitation. The hospital currently has 408 beds, of which 63 are for women, across 22 specialist wards. Approximately 70% of the patients have a diagnosis of mental illness, the remainder having either a personality disorder or a dual diagnosis (mental illness and personality disorder).

Patients admitted to Broadmoor Hospital may be detained under the Mental Health Act (1983), the Crime (Sentences) Act (1997) or the Criminal Procedures (Insanity and Unfitness to Plead) Act (1991) and, again, must be of sufficient risk (to themselves or others) to require conditions of high security. Over half are referred directly from the criminal justice system, the remainder transferring from other National Health Service (NHS) hospitals. The average stay in Broadmoor is eight years, although the length of stay of a patient can be as short as a few months for assessment of suitability for treatment. Or it may be a lifetime for a small number of those who are still considered to be dangerous or who present as treatment resistant. Most patients are transferred out of Broadmoor Hospital to medium secure units. Some are returned to prison and a small number are transferred to conditions of lesser security under supervision.

Broadmoor Hospital plays a pivotal role in carrying out the business of caring for those who pose a threat to society. The management of those threats, or the risk which they present, is core to the success of that aspect of the business. There is an ever-present tension between the needs of individual patients and their rehabilitation and the need for the public to be protected from their potential to cause harm. The perception of risk by the general public has to be recognized as different to the perception of the professional. 'What is risk to the professional is danger to the general public' (Franey and Kaye 1998 p.15).

Broadmoor Hospital and the National Health Service

Broadmoor Hospital became part of the NHS in 1948 and was managed for many years by the Department of Health. In 1988 a highly critical Health Advisory Service (HAS) report was published maintaining that the English high secure hospitals were too 'inward looking' and custodial and made the recommendation that drastic change was required or the hospitals should be closed down (Health Advisory Service 1988). By 1989, Broadmoor was managed by a new body set up by the government – the Special Hospitals Service Authority (SHSA). Not long after, in 1996, the government abolished the SHSA in favour of a similar purchaser/provider environment in keeping with the rest of the NHS. Thus the High Secure Psychiatric Commissioning Board (HSPCB) was set up acting as purchaser and provider of all levels of secure mental health services.

Recent governments have also been committed to a continued modernization of the NHS, and mental health services have become a priority for improvement. High secure hospitals have historically always been isolated from mainstream NHS services. This isolation has been professional, organizational, cultural and geographical. High secure services are challenging because of the types of patients they care for, the need to provide a therapeutic environment while maintaining high levels of security, and because of the stigma that surrounds them (Bacon 2000). The isolation of the high secure psychiatric hospitals from the mainstream NHS not only reduced their capacity to provide the same high-quality services but also led to difficulties in placing patients in the most appropriate level of security while remaining as close to their home as possible.

In 2000, the Government put in place legislative changes that allowed high secure psychiatric services to be managed as part of NHS trusts. The Secretary of State for Health then gave permission for Broadmoor Hospital Authority and Ealing, Hammersmith and Fulham Mental Health NHS Trust to consult publicly on a proposal to establish a single, new organization to provide a full range of local, specialist and forensic mental health services (Bacon 2000).

The formation of this new organization in April 2001, the West London Mental Health NHS Trust was in line with the Government's modernization programme and the National Service Framework (Department of Health 2000b), which set out what users, carers and the public can expect from the NHS and Social Services. The new organizational arrangements aim to ensure that patients who need to be cared for within secure services are more likely to receive a service appropriate to their needs, offering clearer clinical pathways, risk management and concise treatment opportunities.

The occupational therapy and rehabilitation services

Broadmoor Hospital received its first patients in May 1863. A complete community and mostly self-sufficient, the ground plan of the hospital was based on two enclosures: fourteen acres for men and three and half acres for women, with an additional 170 acres of farmland.

A Victorian work ethos provided a utilitarian approach to daily occupations. Facilities included a bakery, laundry, bookbinding, tailors and farm. The gardens and greenhouses were specifically developed for the purpose of growing fruit and vegetables; workshops provided patients with clothing and footwear, the carpenters workshops designed, manufactured and repaired cupboards, bookcases and so on (Goswell 1984).

In 1874, patients began to receive payment for the work they did, instead of being rewarded with beer and cheese, as had initially been the practice. The Rehabilitation Therapy Services (RTS) (formerly known as the Occupations Department) grew out of this ethos. It was underpinned in 1956 by a report of the Committee of Inquiry on the Rehabilitation, Training and Resettlement of Disabled Persons, known also as the *Piercey Report* (1956). This identified the requirement to provide, in the hospital setting if necessary, 'employment, training and occupation for mental patients and defectives of varying grade'.

The modern Occupational Therapy and Rehabilitation Services (OT&RS) has undergone rapid and extensive change over recent years, in line with developments elsewhere in the hospital. Technical instructors (occupations staff) were traditionally recruited from a variety of trade-related backgrounds, and they assisted patients to acquire high levels of skills, as well as providing a service in terms of quality and productivity. This pure-work ethos is no longer appropriate to the current therapy-focused requirements, and today many of the technical instructors continue to have a trade background to which they have added thera-peutic skills and qualifications.

The Occupational Therapy and Rehabilitation Services is composed of four distinct sections:

• Vocational Services
• Sports and Leisure
• Arts Therapies
• Occupational Therapy Services.

The Vocational Services continue to offer trade-orientated activities with opportunities for patients to gain vocational qualifications, for example City and Guilds and NVQs in horticulture and 'real' work experiences. The Sports and Leisure Services aims to provide a calendar of sports, leisure and social events, and the Arts Therapies Service provides music, drama and art therapies. There is also a robust and rapidly expanding Occupational Therapy Service.

The occupational therapy service

Occupational therapists were introduced to Broadmoor Hospital in 1991 following a comprehensive review of the Occupations Department, facili-tated by a newly appointed Director of Rehabilitation Services who herself was an occupational therapist. Since then, seven technical instructors have trained to be occupational therapists and occupational therapy has evolved into a highly specialized service, with an occupational therapist attached to most clinical teams throughout the hospital.

Occupational therapists work alongside technical instructors and provide the knowledge base underpinning much of their joint work together. While the technical instructors provide much of the 'hands on' expertise with regard to arts and crafts and trades, occupational therapists complement these skills by focusing on clinical assessments and treatment interventions to incorporate purpose and meaning for the patients in order to address their needs via relevant activities. The occupational therapist may, for example, use an art and craft group as a medium in which to assess and improve a patient's concentration, communication, social interaction, confidence and self-esteem. The occupational therapist is thus able to articulate more detailed information to clinical teams regarding patient progress, in line with the requirements of the Care Programme Approach.

The philosophy of the occupational therapy service is guided by a patient-centred approach, incorporating the theoretical Model of Human Occupation (Kielhofner 2002) and a problem/asset-oriented system to influence the assessment pathway. A number of standardized assessments are utilized including: Assessment of Occupational Functioning (AOF), the Assessment of Communication and Interaction Skills (ACIS), (Forsyth et al. 1999), the Volitional Questionnaire (VQ) (Chern et al. 1996), the Occupational Self-Assessment (OSA) (Baron et al. 2002) and the Assessment of Motor and Process Skills (AMPS) (Fisher 1999). The choice of assessments used by each occupational therapist varies according to the nature of the patient population and to the needs of the individual patients themselves.

The occupational therapy role in the admissions assessment process

Unlike the other high-security hospitals, Broadmoor Hospital has designated male and female admission wards. The vast majority of patients have come through the criminal justice system, most commonly under Part III of the Mental Health Act (1983) either for pre-trial assessment from court (Sections 35, 38) or for urgent treatment (Sections 48/49) or post-sentencing for assessment and treatment (Sections 47/49). The remainder are admitted from other sources, particularly regional secure facilities (Section 2, Section 3, Section 37 and Sections 37/41).

The multidisciplinary admission case conference takes place three months after admission, marking the end of the assessment process. This is the key decision-making forum where each discipline presents its assessments, followed by a debate in which the initial focus is on consideration of the basic questions posed by the mental health legislation:

- Does this patient have a recognized mental disorder?
- Do they require treatment in hospital?

- Can they be considered treatable?
- Is it necessary that such treatment be carried out in conditions of high security?

If the decision is reached to admit the patient, such issues as initial treatment needs, suitable ward placement and referrals to appropriate disciplines are then discussed.

The assessment process includes objective and subjective information on the patient's current level of occupational functioning and behaviour in the domains of instrumental activities and activities of daily living, these include psychosocial, cognitive, sensorimotor, risk assessment/management and mental state.

Subsequent to an occupational therapy initial interview held on the admissions ward soon after admission, each patient has a set of identified individual assessment aims and objectives and a clear risk-management plan. This is based on the interview and through discussion at weekly multidisciplinary team meetings. A comprehensive documented set of needs is thus present prior to commencing an occupational therapy admissions assessment. The patients are offered a minimum of 30 occupational therapy sessions, pre-case conference, in a variety of settings. These include participating in a wide spectrum of creative task-based activities, discussion groups, sports and leisure activities and cooking sessions. Again, it is this engagement in specific tasks and activities that enables the occupational therapist to assess specific components of an individual's functioning and plan appropriate therapeutic programmes based on any needs identified and also using the patient's identified strengths. Activities can be assigned to the patient that will involve the use of specific skills that can then be assessed. For example, in cooking a simple meal, the occupational therapist can make assessments of cognitive functioning including memory, concentration, ability to follow written or oral instructions, etc. The occupational therapist will also be able to assess the patient's abilities to make decisions independently, deal with problems, their tolerance to frustration and any risks they may present in that situation. The assessment process is guided through the use of clinical pathways, which record each stage and intervention the patient and their occupational therapist have reached.

Some of the key roles of the occupational therapist in the admissions multidisciplinary team include assessing individual occupational performance and task group function related to activities of daily living (basic living skills including self-care, cooking, budgeting, etc. and intrapersonal skills such as problem-solving and coping skills, communication and self-esteem). The occupational therapist also contributes to the diagnosis, risk assessment and management of the patient, and provision of educational resources to students, colleagues and other healthcare professionals.

Occupational therapy and the clinical pathway

Following their admission assessment period, it was not uncommon for Broadmoor patients to transfer to a mainstream ward and lose most, if not all, contact with regular therapies and structured treatment strategies. Emphasis in the past was very much an insistence on patient attendance at RTS 'work' areas to get them off the ward, rather than with the acknowledgement of any therapeutic benefits. This period (often lasting many years) was seen as a time of 'maintenance' until the patient was deemed fit to progress to the pre-discharge wards and thus prepare for eventual transfer.

The resulting lack of therapeutic input and an almost stagnant existence over the years led to a body of men and women becoming highly institutionalized. They are unable to demonstrate realistic survival skills in critical areas such as problem-solving, impulse control and cognitive functioning. They exhibit a parallel decrease in awareness of many basic daily living skills. Self-esteem and confidence are also markedly poor, with some patients refusing to leave the ward environment as a result. There was little or no consistent coordination of a patient's progress throughout the service. In part, this was due to the sheer size and spread of Broadmoor and difficulties in central information gathering. Additionally, it was due to the absence of an identified link person responsible for implementing and coordinating individual patient activity programmes.

Occupational therapy, overall, is playing a key role in redeveloping and maintaining the existing skills of patients who have been in Broadmoor for some time. The occupational therapy clinical pathway also ensures that opportunities for skill maintenance and access to occupational therapy continue. This is part of an ongoing, needs-led, treatment plan once patients have moved on from the admissions assessment ward, helping to avoid the risk of patients becoming swallowed up in the system and perhaps forgotten again. Comprehensive data-collection systems, in the form of an in-house devised structured activity monitoring package, now assist occupational therapists in charting a patient's progress through the system. This system also helps to demonstrate the input offered by occupational therapists to patients.

It may interest the reader to know that while in Broadmoor patients do not have access to cash unless on outside rehabilitation trips, hence patients who are not eligible for these trips may not recognize modern units of currency. A patient on the women's Special Care ward has not boiled a kettle in over eight years, such are the security constraints. But all the more important is the value of promoting the necessity in maintaining even the most basic and fundamental of functional living skills.

Occupational therapists working on the pre-discharge wards have their own set of challenges in preparing patients for transfer to conditions of

lesser security. The pre-discharge wards are generally very quiet and settled wards that admit patients who meet the criteria to maintain this
environmental stability and tranquillity. The difficulty, however, comes
when these very stable and settled individuals are transferred to conditions of lesser security and usually on to an acute admissions ward. One
patient who recently left Broadmoor reported that his belt, shoelaces and
lighter had been removed from him on admission to a medium secure
unit – despite having had all these items for many years prior to his transfer out of Broadmoor. Preparing an individual for this drastic change in
lifestyle is no easy task. Occupational therapists, along with the patient's
clinical team, have a vital role in communicating with recipient agencies
to ensure that the patient is admitted into the appropriate level of care,
taking into account security and clinical needs.

Additional difficulties and uncertainties can also arise at this stage in a
patient's stay in a high secure hospital. A national shortage of medium
secure beds means that a patient can remain within the high secure pre-
discharge services for up to two years, even after the offer of a bed has
been made by a less secure facility. Occupational therapy skills in maintaining motivation and optimism are invaluable at this stage, and a
proactive programme of activities will take these needs into account.

Because high secure environments are comparatively 'resource rich'
environments with high staffing numbers, patients preparing for transfer
or discharge also need to be assisted in developing the skills to cope with
what could be perceived as a less supportive and nurturing environment.

The inability to cope with changes in security levels is frequently evident
within the high secure hospital itself, where choice and individual personal responsibility are removed. Patients moving from higher staffed special
care and admission wards with rigid and structured routines, and optimum levels of security, often experience difficulties settling into more
relaxed regimes on larger wards with lower staffing numbers.
Institutionalization is a daily issue for occupational therapists, who also
aim to help patients relearn to take responsibility for themselves. Again,
this is not an easy task in a high secure environment, which often contra-
dicts occupational therapy philosophies of holistic care and independent
functioning incorporating individual choice. On many of the wards, for
example, patients have restricted access to the bathrooms, which are normally kept locked, limiting their opportunities and choice in personal care
activities. Similarly, ward kitchens are often out of bounds to patients, who
are then dependent on staff for provision of simple liquid refreshment.

Occupational therapists have also been instrumental in addressing the
use of time, encouraging purposeful occupation in work and leisure for
patients, and raising an awareness of quality-of-life issues, particularly
for those patients who are unlikely ever to be released back into the
community.

Women's services

For many years the services provided to women in secure mental health settings have been the subject of much debate, and there is growing acknowledgement that psychiatric services for women, overall, are inferior to those provided for men. A literature review of women and secure psychiatric services (Lart et al. 1999) describes two principal types of services where women's needs appeared to be addressed as either 'an afterthought' or within services that were 'gender blind'.

Women's needs have been consistently neglected, and little effort has been made to take their views into account. It is also widely acknowledged that the majority of women detained in high secure care do not require this level of security. This has never been more evident than at the present time with the implementation of recommendations from the *Tilt Report* (Department of Health 2000a). Broadmoor Hospital is required under the terms of Tilt to provide environmental security equivalent to that of a male category B prison, which is higher than that of a women's category B prison.

Service responses also need to reflect the different experiences and needs of men and women. In line with the national agenda, occupational therapists working in the women's directorate have been instrumental in ensuring the safe provision of services for women patients and in addressing appropriate clinical needs. Issues affecting women in secure care are discussed more widely in Chapter 15 of this book.

Security

Working within a high secure setting often presents a dilemma for occupational therapists trying to balance a therapeutic approach with the demands of security. It can be difficult for the occupational therapist with a patient-centred approach, working in high security, balancing the ever-increasing levels of security with therapy to provide a safe, secure but therapeutic environment for both patients and staff.

In February 2000, the *Tilt Report* (Department of Health 2000a) reviewed security at the three English high-security hospitals and recommended 86 separate improvements to physical and procedural security. This report was commissioned in response to the *Report of the Committee of Inquiry into the Personality Disorder Unit at Ashworth Hospital* (The Fallon Inquiry) (Department of Health 1999). The stringent measures imposed following this review have resulted in occupational therapists reconciling increased security restrictions with intervention planning. It is a challenge for occupational therapists to devise imaginative ways of providing opportunities for patients to feel empowered within this setting.

Now all occupational therapists are involved in a range of physical and procedural security routines. These includes: random pat-down searching and metal detecting of patients leaving therapy areas after each session, the escorting of patients to and from units, maintaining communication through hand-held radios with a central control department, testing and responding to incident alarm bells, searching of units on a weekly and quarterly basis to locate possible weapons or illegal substances and participating in breakaway and control-and-restraint procedures to manage physical aggression.

To ensure security, it is essential that effective communications occur on a daily basis with multidisciplinary teams and nursing teams. Communication and risk assessment are integral factors when planning therapeutic activities. Vital considerations in planning interventions include fluctuating mental states, gender mix, staff:patient ratios and the individual patient's level of safe access to tools and equipment.

Conclusion

It is clear that the roles and skills of the occupational therapist in the high secure setting are unique and diverse. A range of creative and imaginative techniques is required to be employed daily by the therapist in order to optimize therapeutic provision within an environment so dominated by security concerns and occupational deprivation. The occupational therapist needs to reconcile the maintenance of safety and security alongside sustaining the therapeutic relationship between clinician and patient. Within the multidisciplinary setting, occupational therapy can help to promote patient-focused programmes of care and intervention.

The integration of Broadmoor Hospital Authority into the new West London Mental Health NHS Trust (which also incorporates medium and low secure services) offers opportunities for occupational therapists to have experience in a variety of settings. This can be facilitated through rotations and secondments, which also help to avoid burnout and other potentially negative effects that can be encountered when working in a high secure setting. Additionally, it encourages an outward-looking service equal to the high standards of intervention and care expected elsewhere in the NHS.

References

Bacon J (2000) The Establishment of a Mental Health Trust Comprising Broadmoor Hospital Authority and Ealing, Hammersmith and Fulham Mental Health NHS Trust, Consultation Document. Leeds: NHS Executive.

Baron K, Kielhofner G, Iyenger A, Goldhammer V and Wolenski J (2002) A Users Manual for the Occupational Self-Assessment (OSA) (Version 2.0). Chicago: University of Illinois.

Crime Sentences Act (1997) Chapter 43. London: HMSO.

Chern J, Kielhofner G, de las Heras C and Magalhaes L (1996) The volitional questionnaire: Psychometric development and practical use. American Journal of Occupational Therapy 50(7) 516–525.

Criminal Procedures (Insanity and Unfitness to Plead) Act (1991) Chapter 25. London: HMSO.

Department of Health (1999) Executive Summary of the Report of the Committee of Inquiry into the Personality Disorder Unit, Ashworth Special Hospital, chaired by Peter Fallon, QC. London: The Stationery Office.

Department of Health (2000a) Report of the Review of Security at the High Security Hospitals, chaired by Sir Richard Tilt. London: The Stationery Office.

Department of Health (2000b) National Service Framework in Mental Health: Modern Standards and Service Models. London: Department of Health.

Directors of Rehabilitation (1992) Review of the Occupations Service. London: Special Hospitals Service Authority.

Fisher A (1999) The Assessment of Motor and Process Skills. Colorado: Three Star Press.

Forsyth K, Lai J and Kielhofner G (1999) The assessment of communication and interaction skills (ACIS): Measurement properties. British Journal of Occupational Therapy 62(2) 69–74.

Franey A and Kaye C (1998) Managing High Security Psychiatric Care. London: Jessica Kingsley Publishers, Athenaeum.

Goswell B (1984) Work Therapy at Broadmoor. *New Windows*. Staff newspaper of the Department of Health and Social Security. February: 9–10.

Health Advisory Service (1988) HAS Report on Broadmoor Hospital. London: Health Advisory Service.

Kielhofner G (ed.) (2002) A Model of Human Occupation: Theory and Application (3rd edition). Baltimore: Williams and Wilkins.

Lart R, Payne S, Beaumont B, MacDonald G and Mistry T (1999) Women and Secure Psychiatric Services: A Literature Review. York: NHS Centre for Reviews and Dissemination.

Mental Health Act (1959) London: HMSO.

Mental Health Act (1983) London: HMSO.

Piercey Report (1956) Report of a Committee of Inquiry on the Rehabilitation, Training and Resettlement of Disabled People. London: HMSO.

CHAPTER 10

The occupational therapist working in prison

REBECCA HILLS

Introduction

> Good healthcare and health promotion in prisons should help enable individuals to function to their maximum potential on release which may assist in reducing offending.
>
> (HM Prison Service and NHS Executive 1999 p.1)

The development of healthcare provision within the prison service over the past decade has led the service to the point where the aim is now to offer services to prisoners that equal those they would receive as members of the wider community. This development has created the opportunity for occupational therapy to establish its role within the prison system alongside medicine, nursing and psychology. The unique role of the occupational therapist is the ability to address the shift from occupational deprivation to occupational enrichment (Molineux and Whiteford 1999) within such environments. The skills of the occupational therapist include promoting well-being through developing a sense of purpose, enabling the constructive use of energy and time and the acquisition of skills. Thus, it offers prisoners opportunities that are complementary to those offered by other professions and which seek to address the very specific nature of their difficulties.

The development of integrated treatment services for mentally disordered offenders has seen an increase in the numbers of occupational therapists working within all levels of security and within all environments in which the client group receive treatment. Prisons are no exception. Occupational therapists are now working within 18 prisons across the United Kingdom (College of Occupational Therapists 1998) using a variety of treatment models. The addition of occupational therapy provision within the prison service has enabled the profession to provide continuity of care within a truly integrative model. Therefore, a client is able to participate in an occupational therapy programme while in prison, high, medium and low security hospital, hostel and the community. Within this framework the therapist is able to develop a programme of treatment that addresses both the client's needs within the specific environment and which has the potential to be adapted by the therapist, within the receiving service, on transfer.

The development of prison healthcare services

Prison healthcare services within the United Kingdom have, in common with health services in general, been going through an evolutionary process over many years. This process is a useful starting point for the occupational therapist working within the prison environment as it provides a baseline against which a rough gauge of services may be measured. It also allows the occupational therapist to understand the stage of development of healthcare within the prison service as a contrast to the development of general health services.

The UKCC study of nursing practice within secure environments (UKCC 1999) describes the development of the role of specialist 'medical' practitioners (initially doctors) being established as early as 1895 in the prison system. However, it is only since the early 1990s that the aim to ensure prisoners receive 'an equivalent standard of care to that provided by the NHS' (HM Prison Service and NHS Executive 1999) has been expressed. This point has been reached by way of a gradual process – the following documents provide greater detail of this process:

1990 – Efficiency Scrutiny of the Prison Medical Service (Home Office)
1996 – Patient or Prisoner – discussion paper published (HM Inspectorate of Prisons)
1997 – The Provision of Mental Healthcare in prisons (Health Advisory Committee)

These led to:
1999 – The Future Organisation of Prison Health Care (HM Prison Service and NHS Executive)

This last report represented the development of, what were in many respects, radical changes within the provision and organization of prison health services. Its fundamental recommendation was that 'a prison service NHS partnership at all levels is the most practicable way of delivering equivalence of healthcare to the prisoner' (HM Prison Service and NHS Executive 1999 p.42). For the occupational therapist like other health professionals, this report provides a springboard from which to develop services that effectively meet the needs of prisoners. It has also promoted the development of partnerships between prisons and local specialist providers of forensic mental healthcare (Bexley and Greenwich Health Authority, HMP Belmarsh and Oxleas NHS Trust 2000).

Thus, professional standards already established within NHS occupational therapy services may be introduced to healthcare within the prison addressing many quality-of-care issues. This approach enables practitioners to meet the standards expected of them by clinical governance (NHS Executive 1999) including clinical supervision and continuing professional development. It also stimulates the sharing of best practice with colleagues working in similar environments, for example in the development of assessment and intervention systems for the prisoners.

The effect of imprisonment on the individual

> Occupational deprivation is, in essence, a state in which a person or group of people are unable to do what is necessary and meaningful in their lives due to external restrictions. It is a state in which the opportunity to perform those occupations that have social, cultural and personal relevance is rendered difficult if not impossible.
>
> (Whiteford 2000 p.200)

If occupation is considered the process of living our lives (Townsend 1997), imprisonment can be seen as an externally imposed system that inhibits the individual's ability to perform occupation. This creates occupational deprivation, a state where the ability to choose to use a skill or carry out a chosen task is limited by the imposition of external restrictions on the individual over an extensive period of time. Without 'supportive conditions' (Whiteford 2000 p.201), this may lead to occupational dysfunction. It is the ability to analyse the occupational and environmental factors affecting the individual that enables the therapist to develop programmes for intervention to address these issues.

To consider the potential effect of imprisonment upon the individual it is first essential to understand the environment and regimes in which he or she is living, and the type of difficulties faced. Many prisoners are restricted in carrying out personal care activities. They may have to request the use of such items as a razor. They may be observed during personal care activities like showering and toileting. Indeed, they may have restricted access to these facilities. They are likely to have a routine imposed upon them, which may or may not include activities such as work (dependent upon the availability of such roles within the establishment). They may have their meals prepared for them and provided at specified times. Visits from friends or family will invariably be restricted and carried out within a closely monitored environment, as will telephone calls.

Materials, equipment and personal possessions from the world outside of the prison will be again monitored and restricted. Exercise and leisure activities will be provided at a time when members of staff are available to facilitate such activities and conducted within the restrictions imposed by the specific establishment. 'It can seldom be said that the time an inmate spends incarcerated is constructive' (Lloyd 1995 p.21). The day-to-day routines of prison life may be extremely limited. Whiteford (1997 p.127) describes a study of the occupational needs of a group of prisoners in New Zealand where it was noted that there were limited 'activities or rituals to punctuate the passing of the time of day'. This led to such similarity between each day that it had become difficult for the prisoners to retain awareness of the day of the week or indeed the month of the year. The paucity of available cues to guide differentiation of days of the week increases the level of dependency and therefore the level of deprivation for the individual.

The restricted and institutional nature of prison life is by intent not a democratic system. As far as the prisoner is concerned, this lack of opportunity to collaborate or to work in partnership with those who maintain power within the hierarchy presents an inhibitor to the individual's vision of 'hope and possibility of what ought to be or what might be' (Townsend 1997 p.22). It limits the individual's constructive goal-setting potential.

Alongside the deprivation presented by imprisonment, the individual may also have to address an alien subculture, particularly if they are a first-time offender. Within the prison system violence is commonplace often provoked by racial, cultural or sexual tensions (Lloyd 1995). Bullying, harassment and exploitative relationships are additional difficulties to which the individual has to adapt.

Finally, within the prison population there are additional issues related to the health needs of individuals. These may not necessarily be a direct result of imprisonment. Prisoners may present with a mental illness, which has previously been diagnosed and requires ongoing treatment, they may experience stress and anxiety due to the offence and imprisonment, or they may develop a mental illness while in prison. The risk of a prisoner attempting suicide or carrying out self-harm is high. The prison service states that around 1,000 prisoners (of a total prison population in England and Wales of 66,000) are identified as being at risk of self-harm on any given day (HM Prison Service 2001). An increasing number may present with a variety of symptoms and may be defined as having a personality disorder. There are estimated to be approximately 2,000 people thought to have dangerous and severe personality disorder. 'At any time most are in prison or in secure hospitals' (Home Office 1999 p.3). A health needs analysis of a London prison with 703 inmates at the time of the study demonstrated that 550 new patients were seen by the mental health team annually (Bexley and Greenwich Health Authority, HMP Belmarsh and Oxleas NHS Trust 2000). The same report describes the physical conditions for which medication was prescribed during one month as being epilepsy, heart disease, diabetes and asthma. Additionally, many prisoners present with alcohol and drug addictions.

Developing approaches to occupational therapy intervention

Investigation into the work of occupational therapists working within prisons across the United Kingdom demonstrates a variety of approaches. The majority of therapists are providing services as part of a contract with a local NHS service provider, many of these being local forensic or secure services (College of Occupational Therapists 1998). This relationship allows therapists to maintain external professional contacts within the NHS Trust (often clinical supervision and peer support and supervision). It allows them to develop or extend the use of specific models of practice (for example the Model of Human Occupation) into the prison. Additionally, they can transfer NHS methods of developing and maintaining quality services into their work with prisoners. Many therapists provide both individual and group interventions most frequently to those with mental health and emotional difficulties and those presenting with self-harming behaviour (College of Occupational Therapists 1998). Most therapists are employed by mental health trusts and therefore work primarily with prisoners who present with mental health problems. However, occupational therapists with their dual training are additionally able to provide a therapy service for those prisoners with physical problems with the support (and advice) of colleagues with specialist knowledge in the relevant clinical field.

The role of the occupational therapist specializing in mental health in prisons may encompass a number of different areas of skill. A study of the occupational science literature suggests that addressing the problems raised by occupational deprivation should be the therapist's primary role. However, most prisons, particularly training establishments, have workshops, work roles and limited-routine day-to-day activities within the restrictions of prison life. Yet, as discussed earlier, many prisoners may experience occupational deprivation. Molineux and Whiteford (1999) describe this as being the result of the imposition of activities upon the prisoner. The essential ingredient that is missing within this structure is autonomy or choice. Prisoners are often unable to make anything other than limited choices for themselves. Whiteford (1997 p.129) describes the concept of the individual as having 'an internalized vision or picture in your mind and the need to bring that into being'. The need to promote the individual's autonomy and therefore to be able to bring their 'picture into being' provides the therapist with a useful underlying aim for practice.

With this, and the aim of developing individualized treatment pro-grammes guiding the therapist, the method of providing therapeutic programmes may vary. An occupational therapist who works as a lone practitioner may find developing an assessment-based service the most practicable. However, within several prisons across the United Kingdom services are now being developed that allow the therapist (and, indeed, the mental health team) to work within a more familiar framework, that of the community mental health team. Within this framework the therap-ist may work either as a practitioner offering 'outreach' individual services to the community patient (i.e. the prisoner on main location within the prison community) or as a day service provider or both.

Day services within prisons (as in the wider community) provide the dual benefits of enabling the therapist to work with the prisoner to reduce the necessity of admission to 'hospital' (the healthcare centre) or to ease the transition from hospital in-patient to normal location (Nicholls et al. 2001). The Chief Inspector of Prisons commented on such a service in a report into the working of HMP Belmarsh in 1999 saying, 'I must commend the development of the Cass Occupational Therapy Unit. Day care centres are one of the acknowledged ways to help the mentally dis-ordered, those with learning disabilities and others who find difficulty in coping with the demands of every day living' (HM Inspectorate of Prisons 2000 p. 4).

Within the community mental health team and day service structure, the occupational therapist is able to address both lack of choice and occu-pational deprivation while giving close thought to the environment and the development of routines and roles within it. This can occur alongside the development of activity-based programmes that enable assessment of the individual and their needs. The establishment of a close working rela-tionship with the prison discipline staff who manage the prisoner while they are on main location (or in the prison community) enables the ther-apist to develop a potential follow-through to therapeutic work initiated within the day service environment.

Occupational therapy on the Cass Unit, HMP Belmarsh

Occupational therapy at the Cass Unit demonstrates the use of theories that underpin occupational science. Rebeiro and Cook (1999), for ex-ample, identify from their research four stages that group members would experience to achieve occupational functioning in their Conceptual Model of Occupational Spin Off (Rebeiro and Cook 1999 p.184). The first two of these, affirmation (the creation of a warm, accepting and enabling en-vironment) and confirmation (the process of actively engaging in occupations of choice, gaining mastery and realizing accomplishments), are achieved through the facilitation of a needs-led day programme. This enables the prisoners to choose occupations, gain mastery and review their own development within an environment where their views are actively sought and responded to. The final two stages, actualization and anticipation, may be viewed as valuable goals in specific groups of prisoners (an example perhaps being the lifer group). In this way the prisoner who may, for example, be experiencing difficulty coping, be low in mood or unable to manage anger internally is able to develop relevant skills. The use of the day programme and access to individual reviews of need with an identified therapist enables the prisoner to work towards a state of 'Occupational Spin Off' (Rebeiro and Cook 1999 p.184) where they actively seek out other occupations in order to sustain subjective well-being. Within this model the day service may act as a precursor to the prisoner being able to use the wider facilities of the prison programme (workshops, education, sport and exercise, substance misuse programmes, etc.).

The day-care programme within any service should be needs driven and therefore will change frequently over time. Examples of activities or group work used at the Cass Unit include:

- community meetings
- discussion groups
- cognitive-based group work (e.g. mood management, coping skills and assertiveness skills)
- education (literacy, numeracy and information technology)
- stress management/relaxation
- project work (team/group planning)
- art
- music
- art therapy, drama therapy, music therapy
- skills development programmes (e.g. food hygiene)
- creative writing
- leisure activities (e.g. video discussion).

Summary

The relationship between the NHS and the prison service has developed, and the aim now is for prisoners to have equal access to the same standards of healthcare experienced by the wider community. This provides occupational therapy with a unique opportunity to establish a role within this specialist area of healthcare. The development of occupational therapy in prison services includes establishing evidence of its efficacy both in treating the mentally ill offender and, additionally, establishing through research its ability to address offending behaviour.

Most current research on occupational therapy in prisons emanates from New Zealand, Australia or the United States. The effect of imprisonment upon the individual may result in a range of difficulties, which may be identified as occupational deprivation. The therapist can facilitate change in the individual prisoner's occupational functioning by using a range of therapeutic skills.

A community mental health team model (including a day programme) within a carefully planned environment provides a framework for practice. By utilizing knowledge of occupational science, the therapist is able to make a significant impact upon the therapeutic value of prison healthcare.

References

Bexley and Greenwich Health Authority, HMP Belmarsh and Oxleas NHS Trust (2000) Health Needs Assessment. HMP Belmarsh January 2000 (unpublished).

College of Occupational Therapists (1998) Occupational Therapy in Prisons. Report of the study day held at the College of Occupational Therapists on 2 December 1998. London: College of Occupational Therapists.

Health Advisory Committee (1997) The Provision of Mental Health Care in Prisons. HMP Prison Service. London: HMSO.

HM Inspectorate of Prisons (1996) Patient or Prisoner? A New strategy for health care in prisons. London: Home Office Publications.

HM Inspectorate of Prisons (2000) Report of Inspectorate Visit to HMP Belmarsh December 1999. London: HM Inspectorate of Prisons.

HM Prison Service and NHS Executive (1999) The Future Organisation of Prison Healthcare. London: Department of Health.

HM Prison Service (2001) Prevention of Suicide and Self-harm in the Prison Service. London: HM Prison Service.

Home Office (1990) Report on an Efficiency Scrutiny to the Prison Medical Service. London: Home Office.

Home Office (1999) Managing Dangerous People with Severe Personality Disorder. Proposals for Policy Development. London: Department of Health.

Lloyd C (1995) Forensic Psychiatry for Health Professionals. London: Chapman and Hall.

Molineux M and Whiteford G (1999) Prisons: From occupational deprivation to occupational enrichment. Journal of Occupational Science 6(3) 124–130.

NHS Executive (1999) Clinical Governance Quality in the New NHS. Leeds: Department of Health.

Nicholls T, Czajkowski J and Hills R (2001) The Cass Unit Annual Review 2001. Oxleas NHS Trust (unpublished).

Rebeiro K and Cook J (1999) Opportunity, not prescription: An exploratory study of the experience of occupational engagement. Canadian Journal of Occupational Therapy 66(4) 176–187.

Townsend E (1997) Occupation: Potential for personal and social transformation. Journal of Occupational Science 4(1) 18–26.

CHAPTER 11

The development of community forensic occupational therapy

CATHERINE JOE

Introduction

The rapidly expanding forensic mental health services have seen the emergence of a new professional role, that of community forensic occupational therapy. Each year, more medium secure units are opening; in addition to this, following the *Tilt Report* (Department of Health 2000) the Government has been making significant changes to the function of the special hospitals in England. One outcome has been to review the levels of security required by each patient. Those who no longer need to be detained within a high secure environment, but continue to need care, may be managed in medium secure settings. It is planned that this group of patients should be relocated to secure units local to their catchment area. Also, the aim now is to place people, at the point of admission to the service, in the minimum level of security necessary. In practice, this means many patients may only use medium secure services. Those who no longer represent an immediate risk will eventually be resettled in the community. The advantages of specialist support for these patients by community forensic mental health teams are being increasingly recognized. This includes an increased understanding of the importance of occupational and social dimensions in restoring and maintaining mental health alongside the more traditional aspects of medication, risk assessment and support.

This chapter considers different frameworks within which community forensic occupational therapy is provided, but focuses particularly on the role of the community forensic occupational therapist working within the community forensic mental health team. In this setting, the therapist is required to work generically (using shared skills and blurring their role with other disciplines) but also to provide specialist interventions. Thus, some aspects of the community forensic mental health team are described here. The nature of the therapeutic relationship is also considered. First, however, attention is given to two key issues influencing community forensic occupational therapy: discrimination and social inclusion.

Discrimination

Individuals who have been through forensic services are discriminated against twice. They not only have a psychiatric label of mental illness or personality disorder, they also have to contend with the implications of being under the care of forensic services. This indicates that they have the complication of offending behaviour and may be dangerous. This can often raise anxiety in community agencies, including their fears of having to manage potential risks. Many agencies are therefore reluctant to accept individuals with forensic histories. 'In addition to suffering stigma related to their illnesses, they find that even treatment is difficult to access due to their criminal histories' (Roskes et al. 1999 p.461). For those patients involved in the criminal justice system, they often face five barriers to care. These are: double stigma, lack of family and social support, co-morbidity problems, problems with adjustment on return to the community, and boundary issues between healthcare and the criminal justice system.

In Britain, 35% of all people classified as disabled (including those with mental health, learning disabilities, physical disabilities and sensory impairments) are working (Department for Education and Employment 1998). Within this group, the rate for people with long-term mental illness who are working is even lower; it is a mere 13%, and for black users and those with criminal records, it is even worse (Sayce 2000a). People who experience mental health problems and are also in forensic services benefit the least from the existing range of work and social opportunities on offer, making them one of the most excluded groups within the community.

Forensic services recognize that care plans for those in their service will be influenced and directed by the risk that service users pose to the public. On the other hand, service users have a right to equitable access to healthcare and treatment. These services should be at the same level that the non-offending mental health population receives.

Social inclusion

Social inclusion recognizes that people who are impeded, or excluded, from contributing to the decisions and services that affect their lives are denied citizenship. Many mental health service users are excluded from citizenship due to the stigmas of mental illness, offending, low levels of education and employability (Millar 2000). The social inclusion of individuals with mental illness may possibly reduce their risk of offending and reduce the damaging social effects of exclusion.

This notion is supported by mental health users' experiences of discrimination (Sayce 2000a). The mental health survivor's movement believes that society should address discriminatory attitudes and make practical adjustments to their workplace routines and the public environment. Although these ideals are supported by the Disability Discrimination Act (1995) and the Disability Rights Commission (Disability Rights Task Force 1999), experience suggests considerable changes are necessary before this is achieved for the forensic patient. In order for individuals who have mental illness to contribute on an equal footing with those who do not have mental illness, adjustments such as working from home, having a quiet work area, receiving extra support and feedback may be necessary. Action on many levels is important, including the use of the media and education to change public attitudes, preventing not-in-my-backyard (nimby) campaigns. Action should also focus on: changing the use of everyday language which denigrates mental illness, changes in the law and policy, use of anti-discrimination law, supporting user/survivor projects, grass-roots work and alliances (Sayce 2000a). Such actions lay the groundwork for acceptance of clients, whether they recover or not, and support individual choices of how people use mental health services.

Frameworks for community forensic occupational therapy provision

Within a forensic service, occupational therapists can provide community sessions in the following ways:

1. **As a member of the community forensic mental health team** An occupational therapist can be employed as a member of a community forensic team where his or her work is based entirely in the community. This provides equity of service in line with community mental health team (CMHT) levels where occupational therapy is a core discipline within the service. In this framework, occupational therapy is available for patients living in all catchment areas and the therapist receives referrals from both outpatient clinics and in-patient units. The patient group includes: those being discharged from secure units into the community, outpatient sex offenders and others with a forensic history who live in the community but need support during an acute period or crisis.

2. **A dedicated post to a specific community resource** An occupational therapist can be employed to work specifically in a community setting such as a forensic or offender hostel. Here the occupational therapist will be responsible for providing structured daytime activities, engaging individuals in community facilities and offering specific interventions as required.

3. **A post split between in-patient services and the community** More commonly, occupational therapists already working within a secure unit provide a few community sessions. Here interventions can include follow-up and support for those discharged from in-patient units, focusing on resettlement into the community. It may also include facilitating specific groups, for example in a sex offender treatment programme.

The community forensic mental health team

A community forensic mental health team can manage their caseload with differing levels of responsibility. They may retain total responsibility for all the supervision and care of forensic clients or they can work jointly with the patient's local CMHT, in a consultancy role, and share these responsibilities. The general mental health services may manage many individuals with forensic histories, when they no longer require the specialist interventions of a forensic team. In order to provide the most appropriate care, and not to detain patients in a secure environment unnecessarily restrictive to their needs, the team will have established networks with the local acute admission units. Those who relapse may need admission only into an open acute admission ward rather than a medium secure ward.

Community forensic teams may use some methods from the model of Assertive Community Treatment (Kent and Burns 1996, Burns and Guest 1999). This is a form of intensive case management. This model is proven to provide effective care to a group of community patients who are characteristically difficult to engage and have severe and enduring mental illness and social problems. Staff members have a smaller caseload compared with a CMHT, and they assertively engage clients by establishing a helpful relationship with frequent contact. The team prioritizes those interventions which have been demonstrated to be effective for this group, such as supervision with medication, early interventions to minimize relapse of illness, maintaining stable accommodation, assisting with household tasks, minimizing social stressors, support for carers and family work.

Community forensic mental health teams are multidisciplinary. Each member, regardless of their professional label, performs functions based on the individual's care plan. It involves assertively establishing a therapeutic relationship with the client, following them into the community and linking them into whatever community resource is most appropriate. However, it may prove ineffective if the community lacks the resources or support required, or if the professional is unable to engage the client (Chaloner and Coffey 2000).

Research on the role of case management has demonstrated that the combination of extended mental health treatment with active case management keeps clients out of jail (Steadman et al. 1995). It can be an appropriate strategy for the management of risk, and it benefits social functioning, improves symptomology, generates greater satisfaction with services, and decreases the family burden and days in hospital. Within the English healthcare system, best-practice principles of intensive case management can be provided under the care programme approach where the staff act as keyworkers (Kent and Burns 1996).

Where occupational therapists act as keyworkers, they may perform many generic duties similar to other professional colleagues. There are advantages and disadvantages to being a keyworker. One advantage is that it meets Prins' (1993) recommendations for managing the potentially dangerous offender patient. He suggests good teamwork, collaboration, a capacity for professionals to cross boundaries and the need to give up territorial traditions are necessary. It can also be particularly valuable for the community forensic occupational therapist to act as keyworker for those individuals where their integration into social networks and community facilities is a priority. In one team, an occupational therapist who did not have a keyworker role felt marginalised by some clients, since her interventions were not perceived by them as a compulsory, and important, part of the care plan. However, a disadvantage of being a keyworker is that the legal issues may distort the relationship. Personal experience suggests clients tend to perceive the nursing role as part of their 'parole' conditions. Whereas occupational therapists are not viewed in this manner so much, because the aim of contact is for specific lifestyle work within a collaborative relationship. This allows the therapist to build a more equal therapeutic relationship based on achieving specific goals.

The role of the community forensic occupational therapist

Important legislation further supports developing the role of the community forensic occupational therapist. The National Service Framework for Mental Health (Department of Health 1999) outlines that clients who are managed under the enhanced care programme approach should receive services in the following areas: employment, education or training, promoting independence and sustaining social contact including therapeutic leisure activity and domestic support provision. All these areas are in the direct professional domain of the occupational therapist.

What distinguishes the occupational therapist who works in a community forensic mental health team from an occupational therapist working in a CMHT within adult services is not their clinical interventions but the requirement to work under a legal framework. Many, but not all, of the individuals on the community forensic occupational therapist's caseload will be subject to restriction orders either through the Home Office or the Probation Service. This may influence or distort the therapeutic relationship. There is also an expectation that treatment and interventions are provided in a way that ensures public safety (Wasyliw and Cavanaugh 1988). Prins (1990) suggests the best approach is to give great attention to detail, to have a high threshold of 'suspiciousness' and a capacity to maintain a level of supervision, which often needs to be more intrusive than in other areas of mental health counselling. Risk issues are frequently concerned with the type of relationships that mentally dis-ordered offenders develop with others and certain behaviours that they may hide from members of the team.

Interventions

The aim of facilitating social inclusion is frequently the primary aim of the occupational therapy treatment plan. Many referrals will often be to facil-itate meaningful day activities for the client in the community in order to provide a daily structure and to develop positive social roles. To do this it is necessary to build up varied networks and relationships with a range of community agencies as well as the usual community mental health ser-vices. These personal contacts are important when introducing forensic clients to a new community venue.

In the choice of placement, the therapist has to consider the balance of ensuring the safety of the public against the client's right of access to opportunities that are equal to other users of health and social services. A poorly chosen placement may increase the risk factors. Examples include where there is easy access to drugs and alcohol, contact with vulnerable women or opportunities for criminal activity. This therapeutic dilemma is common and is often difficult to resolve satisfactorily for occupational therapists. Ultimately, however, the burden of responsibility does not fall to them alone. It is a decision for the whole multidisciplinary team.

One reason to take therapeutic risks is that engagement in appropriate low-risk settings will enable the team to better monitor the client. This may be preferable to excluding the client from activities where they would have little structure or focus and therefore become difficult to monitor. Discrimination and prejudice can block access to many community services, even services that specifically cater for mental health users. Ongoing sup-port may need to be provided to both the client and the staff in the placement. The approach should be to educate and demystify the fears and anxieties staff may have, and prevent any discrimination. For referrals to community vocational and social agencies, the occupational therapist needs to promote a non-prejudicial approach but, at the same time, share relevant information. Providing practical recommendations to minimize risks, and clear specific goals for this intervention, assists both therapist and agency to monitor the client safely and assess their progress in achieving the goals.

Work is an activity that promotes social inclusion for clients. It is valu-able to liaise with organizations that specifically assist in the resettlement of ex-offenders, such as the National Association for the Care and Resettlement of Offenders (NACRO). They have developed expertise and networks in assisting ex-offenders to gain employment, and offer training, job placement and practical advice, such as filling in application forms. In a job application, clients may have to disclose offences and account for a long period in secure facilities. Often clients may have the appropriate work skills and motivation but feel unable to confront the difficulties in dealing with the potential discrimination of employers.

The occupational therapist is often the main person facilitating the client's vocational rehabilitation. The model of Supported Employment (Crowther et al. 2001) has proved to be successful in enabling people to gain and maintain open employment. The model focuses on rapid job-search and minimal pre-vocational training. Employees are provided with ongoing assessment and review, with support for as long as is necessary. The occupational therapist can also support the employer by focusing on the job and dealing with concerns as they arise. There are also more specialist vocational agencies that provide training, job-seeking skills and ongoing support to people with mental health problems. By facilitating clients into training schemes or open employment and developing their coping strategies the occupational therapist contributes towards improving citizen opportunities for them at a grass-roots level.

The resettlement of clients who have lived in an institution for many years presents unique challenges. The behaviours and attitudes apparent during incarceration may continue in the community, and the stressors are frequently significantly greater. During incarceration, individuals will be used to having easy access to many activities, yet they will have had limited responsibility in organizing the structure of their day. On discharge to the community, they are faced with a limited choice of appropriate facilities and will have greater difficulty in accessing them. Consequently, they have to deal with a lack of daily structure and routine. Therefore, discharge needs to be graded, to allow for adjustment and to enable them to establish new relationships and routines.

Occupational therapy interventions can be goal-focused and time-limited. That is, contact ends when the goal is reached, for example with a work placement or on completion of stress management training sessions. The occupational therapist can provide a comprehensive assessment of the client's functioning and devise a programme to promote their strengths as well as providing interventions enabling the client to cope better in their day-to-day life. Detailed use of assessments is covered elsewhere in this book. All interventions aim at enhancing the client's opportunity to live independently in the community. By careful assessment, the client's level of functioning is ascertained. The next important stage is collaborative goal-setting. After an occupational therapy assessment and a team risk assessment, if engagement to a specific community venue is regarded as both beneficial and safe, the therapist will address two distinct aspects. For example, with a work placement, the occupational therapist has a role both with the employer and the employee. With the employer the therapist may need to act as an advocate and, at the same time, give advice on how to adapt the workplace for the client. For the client, that is the employee, the occupational therapist may need to act in the role as a job coach until the individual is settled into a job, as well as providing regular support.

The Psychosocial Interventions model (Birchwood 1999) can be effectively used by the occupational therapist with individuals whose functional problems are caused by a severe and enduring mental illness, as the risk of offending is often related to a relapse of their mental illness. The model focuses on the interaction between exposure to environmental stress and individual vulnerability factors. It uses behavioural and cognitive-behavioural techniques to manage psychosis. It involves the social network and structured family therapy (psycho-education, communication skills training and problem-solving skills). There is research evidence of its effectiveness in the management of schizophrenia if applied in a systematic way (Chaloner and Coffey 2000).

The approach of Psychosocial Interventions is problem-centred; this is potentially in conflict with most occupational therapy models that tend to be client-centred and strengths-focused models. However, both these approaches can work in a complementary way. In order for the client to live as independently as possible, this often means they need to learn to cope with enduring mental health problems and find a way of minimizing the disabling effects of mental illness. Improvements in mental state, social networks and family relationships would enable the individual to more readily achieve the aims of their occupational therapy treatment. Often treatment aims, within each approach, will be similar, such as improving social networks or better management of their stress.

The therapeutic relationship

The forensic caseload often contains a small but significant percentage of individuals who have severe personality problems including some that are potentially dangerous and continue to pose significant risk. In order to establish a good working relationship with this client group, the therapist needs to be highly skilled. Prins (1990) suggests they need to be empathic but without being naïve and able to critically appraise and analyse the client's motivation for treatment. An attitude of openness to address issues in conjunction with the team is required plus an ability to use an assertive community treatment approach where needed. The relationship established with the individual can become distorted due to the legal requirements and the need for all staff to monitor levels of risk. It is important to acknowledge that the legal context and the background of the client can also distort the therapist's attitudes. Wasyliw and

Cavanaugh (1988) identify that therapists' attitudes can be distorted, for example about a patient's potential for violence or about the nature of past criminal acts. A therapist's fear of violence, whether justified or not, may create exaggeration or minimization of actual danger. This may be related to countertransference issues such as the therapist's own unresolved anger, fear of losing control or denial as a defensive reaction. Prins (1990) recommends an attitude of 'ambivalent investment' in dealing with some complex or difficult cases. Clinicians will have to come to terms with their own feelings about the offences that clients have committed. They have to manage the balance of public risk and patient rights. They have to be aware that a high therapeutic investment, and hope of success, does not mean their becoming selective and ignoring more subtle cues. Clinicians have to be perceptive to these subtle nuances in behaviour and to use this knowledge to assist the client in safely addressing frightening thoughts and fantasies, or to confront undesirable or seriously antisocial behaviour.

If the therapist is unable to work through and manage these issues, they will be unable to advocate for the client or provide realistic support. Close teamwork and regular supervision will ensure that good and safe practice takes place so that the therapist is able to provide an equitable service to a challenging client group.

Conclusion

This chapter attempts to link the range of influences in the development of community forensic occupational therapy. Significantly, the core philosophical and professional values of occupational therapy are being increasingly reflected in governmental health aims. There is recognition that social and occupational dimensions are important in the achievement and maintenance of mental health.

The challenges for the therapist are the, often contradictory, goals of social inclusion, treatment and public safety. This requires the occupational therapist to develop specific generic skills as well as the ability to provide specialist interventions and assume specialist roles. There is a need for research into the efficacy of community forensic occupational therapy, particularly its contribution to the integration of forensic clients back into society. Much of the current focus for community forensic patients is on safety and treatment. While these are very important responsibilities, services need also to incorporate the findings from user research. The highest priorities, which users repeatedly identify as the interventions with the greatest health gains, are employment, money and opportunities for social participation (Sayce 2000b). The occupational therapist is a key professional in enabling the individual to achieve these aims.

References

Birchwood M (1999) Psychological and social treatments: Course and outcome. Current Opinion in Psychiatry 12: 61–66.

Burns T and Guest L (1999) Running an assertive community treatment team. Advances in Psychiatric Treatment 5: 348–356.

Chaloner C and Coffey C (eds.) (2000) Forensic Mental Health Nursing: Current Approaches. Oxford: Blackwell Science.

Crowther R, Marshall M, Bond G and Huxley P (2001) Helping people with severe mental illness to obtain work: Systemic review. British Medical Journal 322: 204–208.

Department for Education and Employment (1998) Labour Force Survey 1997/8: Unemployment and Activity Rates for People of Working Age. Background Paper for Welfare to Work Seminar. London: Department for Education and Employment.

Department of Health (1999) National Service Framework for Mental Health, Standards and Service Models. London: Department of Health.

Department of Health (2000) Report of the Review of Security at the High Security Hospitals, Chairman Sir Richard Tilt. London: The Stationery Office.

Disability Rights Act (1995) London: The Stationery Office.

Disability Rights Task Force (1999) From Exclusion to Inclusion. London: Department for Education and Employment.

Kent A and Burns T (1996) Setting up an assertive community treatment service. Advances in Psychiatric Treatment 2: 143–150.

Millar C (2000) Citizenship and inclusion. Open Mind, the Mental Health Magazine 105 (Sept/Oct) 10–11.

Prins H (1990) Supervision of Potentially Dangerous Offender-patients in England and Wales. International Journal of Offender Therapy and Comparative Criminology 34(3) 213–221.

Prins H (1993) Service provision and facilities for the mentally disordered offender. In: Clinical Approaches to the Mentally Disordered Offender, Howells K and Hollin C (eds.). Chichester: John Wiley and Sons.

Roskes E, Felman R, Arrington S and Leister M (1999) A model programme for the treatment of mentally ill offenders in the community. Community Mental Health Journal 35(5) 461–475.

Sayce L (2000a) From Psychiatric Patient to Citizen – Overcoming Discrimination and Social Exclusion. London: Macmillan Press.

Sayce L (2000b) Mainstreaming mental health. Open Mind, the Mental Health Magazine 102 (Mar/Apr) 13.

Steadman H, Morris S and Dennis D (1995) The diversion of mentally ill persons from jails to community-based services: a profile of programs. American Journal of Public Health 85(12) 1630–1635

Wasyliw O and Cavanaugh J (1988) Clinical Considerations in the Community Treatment of Mentally Disordered Offenders. International Journal of Law and Psychiatry 11(4) 371–380.

PART FOUR
SPECIAL ISSUES ARISING

CHAPTER 12
Setting up a forensic occupational therapy service

GILL URQUHART

Introduction

The specialism of forensic healthcare has come of age both within the health and social sectors, and, in the private provider organizations. Nowhere has it gained more of a distinct demarcation than in the mind of the public through high-profile cases such as Christopher Clunis, a schizophrenic man who drew much media attention following the murder of Jonathan Zito (Ritchie et al. 1994). Public interest regarding the role and function of secure settings has brought both positive and negative challenges and has rightly led clinical professions to carefully scrutinize their contributions to this client group.

The State Hospitals Board for Scotland was the first high secure NHS establishment in the United Kingdom to employ occupational therapists in the early 1990s. At this time, this organization was becoming a part of the National Health Service, and the effects on existing staff during this time were significant. Morale was low, demands to change and improve services for patients were high. Yet, as ever, the repercussions of getting things wrong were significant. The consequences of breakdowns in risk assessment and management strategies, and media interest, were then, as they are now, unyielding to the smallest of errors. This first introduction of occupational therapy was not successful and, within the space of approximately four years, all the therapists had left the organization. This apparent failure was a bitter pill for both the profession and the organization to swallow. The decision to reintroduce therapists was to come about some three years later, following a service review conducted by the Scottish Health Advisory Service (1990).

In the intervening years, the hospital had undergone several key changes to its culture and personnel. The hospital's board of management was also clearly focused on the potential contributions that occupational therapists were making in more mainstream mental health and learning disabilities services. In 1997, the then Director of Nursing addressed a focus group, looking at the contributions made by occupational therapy elsewhere to the mentally disordered offender. He concluded that, 'It is essential that the introduction of any services within forensic health is fully supported and integrated from the bottom up, and the top down. And that if it is hoped that the investment of £40,000 and a lick of paint in a Portakabin, somewhere on campus, is a good enough start-up, don't waste your money!'

This chapter describes the stages, pitfalls, and successes of introducing occupational therapy to the State Hospital from 1997 to date. The service is no longer viewed as 'under development'; it has come of age, yet we have succeeded in maintaining its vibrancy along with a sense of moving forward and ongoing consolidation. It is essential to acknowledge the individual contribution made by the various staff, both past and present. Without their determination and skills, it is questionable whether this service would have enjoyed the level of integration that it now does.

Stage 1 – Recognize what type of organization you are entering

Large institutions do have strong cultures and value systems. This may appear obvious; however, successful integration depends on these being understood and handled with care by any newcomers. Interestingly, this statement applies as much to new patients as to new staff, although the effects are clearly different. Goffman (1961) describes how some institutions or establishments could be viewed as 'total institutions'. He uses this term to convey the organization's separateness from the world, the powers of control and containment it exerts over the inhabitants and the unique nature of the work and practices carried out. He describes how residents of total institutions are cut off from wider society for long periods and lead enclosed lives regulated by the organization. In short, a total institution is fully self-sufficient, physically separated from the outside world and requires inhabitants to carry out a full range of human activities within the same place and often in collective groups. Perhaps most significantly, Goffman (1961 p.17) states that in a total institution 'the various enforced activities are brought together into a single rational plan purportedly designed to fulfil the official aims of the institution'. He identifies various organizations as potentials for such a definition, including, amongst others, retreats, prisoner-of-war camps, boarding schools and mental hospitals.

For the purposes of this chapter, it may be reasonable to consider to what extent one can apply the term 'total' whether in whole or part to forensic institutions. Historically, the providers of specialized forensic healthcare were less open to outward, or inward, looking scrutiny and as such were protected from the need to assess their performance against the wider world of healthcare.

Lloyd (1987) discusses the impact of such institutions in greater detail. It is important, when planning services, to recognize the impact on working practices an institution can have on both staff and patients. Over the past decade, with the drive towards clinical effectiveness, clinical governance, accreditation and public scrutiny, much has been achieved to erode the negative consequences of the 'total institution' on patients and on their daily routines. However, there is still much that requires to be done to prevent practices serving the organization's needs, rather than the therapeutic needs of its patients.

During the first weeks and months of 1997, considerable time was spent mindfully clarifying the cultural strengths and weaknesses of the State Hospital from the bottom up, especially where patients' routines were at times unhelpful to their rehabilitation or, at worst, counterproductive. As with any new service development, a guiding principle was that occupational therapy must add clinical value to overall patient care. At this early stage, we were careful not to criticize the current methods of delivering activities to patients, as failure to tread sensitively generally leads to blocking and non-cooperation from colleagues across the organization.

A central issue facing most forensic organizations is in the development of their policies and subsequent staff training on the prevention and management of aggression, the fundamental principles of which are universal. These are: the use of de-escalation techniques, reduction or minimization of risk of harm to all concerned and, most importantly, that physical restraint or control of a patient should be deployed only as a last resort. As with most secure provisions, the issue of who can and should be involved in responding to emergencies was seen solely as the domain of the nursing profession and their support staff. Many excuses were offered explaining why other clinical professions did not at this time assist in the management of aggression. Most often, these explanations were associated with the potentially damaging impact this could have on the therapeutic relationships other professionals had with patients. The occupational therapy view was that simply by choosing to work with patients who are all being legally detained against their will, by definition, immediately produces a potential impediment to therapy. This was something that all staff including nurses had to overcome. No single therapist has ever questioned or disagreed with the decision to undertake the training on aggression management, which was to be a significant factor that helped to cement the interdisciplinary relationships with our colleagues in nursing and allowed the therapists to be more self-sufficient.

Our next decision was on how best to deploy the growing number of therapists around the organization. We had already decided on a clear and defined model of practice, the Model of Human Occupation (MoHO) (Kielhofner 1997). At a very early stage, clarity in the use and application of the model assisted therapists in their day-to-day tasks and interventions. By the summer of 1997, we were ready to place four new therapists into the clinical field.

Stage 2 – Get to know the key people, and get to know your market

The carriers of any institution's culture include representatives from the full spectrum of roles and grades, including corporate decision-makers such as directors and senior managers. Although it may seem unnecessary to spend time listening to their 'storytelling', much can be gained from these insights into both past events and present hopes and aspirations. By investing in these stories, a picture emerges which gives insights into service gaps and how best to place and target any new resources or service developments.

As with many forensic institutions, there were already established daytime occupations for patients. These activities were tightly scheduled at pre-arranged intervals, staffed by nurses and technical support staff. As occupational therapists whose treatment modality is purposeful and meaningful activity, we were aware that focusing on what was already being delivered and introducing modifications in these areas would not have brought the best added value by our introduction. The therapists were keen to develop new options in patient care and to roll out our expertise in assessing and treating patients unable to access what was already present. To date, the needs of those with severe and enduring treatment-resistant mental illness remain our highest priority, as do those with challenging behavioural problems.

We noted our growing alliance with nursing staff and felt that our method of delivering the best services was to place a therapist as part of a core clinical team in each of the then ten wards. Our first business plan was produced, which itemized the additional posts needed for the remainder of the financial year. By the end of the year, we had eight staff in place. We were ready to move into the newly refurbished department, and, although ready to have our first patients into treatment sessions, the therapists continued to carry out ward-based activity sessions with ward-based nurses.

Much time was invested in joint working with named nurses or key-workers, and setting down and developing service standards in line with College of Occupational Therapists guidelines (College of Occupational

Therapists 2001). This work, combined with that of other disciplines, was later to form the basis of multidisciplinary integrated care pathways.

Stage 3 – Our first takeover or merger

The idea of a takeover is fraught with negative connotations, as it implies an imbalance of power and status between one collective and another. However, around the end of the first year, the therapists were asked to consider taking the nurse-led Lifeskills Unit and running it as part of the occupational therapy service. This service had been most closely aligned to core occupational therapy practices. It provided personal and domestic activities of daily living, communications-skills development sessions and social performance sessions amongst others. Based in a separate building and run by nursing and support staff, the Lifeskills Unit was seen as valuable but suffered from a lack of clarity of its aims and methods of achievement. Following the merger, several of the existing staff were redeployed, at their request, to other activity areas not under the occupational therapy umbrella. This allowed a trained occupational therapist to be introduced into the Lifeskills Unit and be based in the same building. However, the ensuing consequences were seen as markers of how far we still had to go to overcome the suspicion of our colleagues who voted with their feet rather than be managed by our service! In an attempt to close this gap we decided to retain the staff-nurse post in the Lifeskills Unit, giving a clear message to nursing colleagues that life skills development is not the sole responsibility of our professional group. It worked!

Stage 4 – Introducing new concepts and new risks

An early concern in the minds of colleagues was the fear that therapists may, either by design or omission, introduce high-risk working practices that would undermine the safety of both patients and staff. In short, the therapists may work in new ways, and divergence from routine practice might be bad! Given that on several occasions the therapists were told that 'you can't work here unless you already have forensic experience', it was important to educate others in our core skills of functional assessment and activity analysis, which applies equally to the forensic field as to mainstream mental health.

As a new group of staff, the learning curve was fast and steep, in order to become expert in thinking through the myriad processes involved in risk assessment and risk management. Unlike new recruits in wards, where the main bodies of staff already have many years of experience, the entire therapist group was learning at the same time and at roughly the same pace. Any mistakes would have raised doubts in the overall competence of the occupational therapy service to manage safety. In response to this, the therapists temporarily became risk aversive until they had learned to become risk managers.

As with many occupational therapy programmes, the therapeutic kitchen was a highly sought-after site for patients to attend. As an example of the new risk management thinking, the kitchen and its safe operating became the focus of many hours of discussion and debate both for us and for clinical teams. Much help and advice was given by colleagues in security and nursing to help the therapists introduce ways of managing the space and tools. The aim was to enable the patients who posed higher risks of self-harm and, in some cases, high risk to others, to access the service. By doing so, the service entered many long hours of hard focused thinking-through of the ethical and practical issues, to find solutions where appropriate and to overcome the risks. In some instances, the solution was simply not to take the risks, as no practical alternative was available at that time. However, even in the early days, solutions often became apparent after debate with the wider clinical teams.

As with many forensic hospitals, a high proportion of our patient group has a primary diagnosis of schizophrenia. At that time, any therapeutic sessions conducted off ward had been in two main blocks, that is either for the morning or the afternoon. Given the difficulties faced by the patient group, and the need to maximize the variety of interventions available, the occupational therapy service pioneered the introduction of tailoring the timing of sessions. These linked with other services and thus offered choice and scope in the patients' overall daily schedule. The challenges of such a change focused mainly on the need for exceptionally high standards of communication with all staff. The organization had now begun to move towards planning activity to meet individuals' needs, rather than moving patients en masse in ways that suited the organization.

Stage 5 – Research and advanced practice: can we do this too?

As with all modern healthcare, clinical research and advanced practices in the forensic field are high priorities, to ensure a growth of clinical evidence that will serve the public-safety agenda. From the outset new services should gather clinical evidence through a structured research programme. Failure to do so results in a lack of evidence to support current or future practices and, at worst, could allow unsound methods to continually be employed by well-meaning professionals.

In the State Hospital the offer of financial support to appoint a research consultant from Queen Margaret's University College in Edinburgh was grasped, and, in recent years, this model has been replicated in other services north and south. The therapists' ability to critically appraise methods and techniques rapidly developed. They are now actively

involved in the process of disseminating their findings through presenting papers at national events and publishing articles. To date, the results
of this investment have been significant, although experience suggests
there is a time lag of approximately 18 months from introducing an academic link before any widespread impact, both internally and externally,
is felt within the organization.

All staff must be encouraged to feel a sense of ownership of the
research agenda and to take responsibility of their own advanced practice.
Various methods are employed to achieve this aim, and include objective
setting, competency management tools and involving staff directly in the
annual business planning process. The model used in the State Hospital
is one of many, but it has been tailored to promote the most cost-effective
impact on all, including qualified and support staff. Regular supervision is
essential and is closely linked to each individual's competence as a
researcher. Should you consider embarking on a link position, a baseline
study into the impact of this type of academic link needs to be considered.

Stage 6 – Retention, not forgetting recruitment

While the shortfall of state registered occupational therapists continues to
be a concern (Department of Health 2000, College of Occupational
Therapists 2000), the value and contribution that therapists have within
forensic services grows. This goes some way to explain the shortfall
between supply and demand (Duncan 1999). Whether wishing to recruit
to a new service, or struggling to recruit to an existing one, the promotion of an organization that values and supports its staff, and is prepared
to invest in them, cannot be emphasized enough. However, on a caution-
ary note, nothing will spread quicker than false promises that are made at
interviews that subsequently cannot be upheld six months down the line!

Recruitment strategies that have been successful in the State Hospital
have included being clear about what the service will offer each new
recruit. Also we targeted the market, that is reaching occupational therapists at conferences, workshops and through written publications. It is
essential to think ahead and plan student placements and visits from
undergraduates. We encourage lectures at local universities by staff and
are careful not to take only final-year students. Many therapists choose to
work in areas where they have had their first positive clinical experience
and have chosen never to work in a field where they had an unhappy
experience, so beware.

The forensic field also carries a speciality label, which can potentially
frighten away possible recruits from more mainstream settings. Ensuring
a steady stream of undergraduates throughout their studies should help
in demystifying some of the preconceived ideas still prevalent regarding

forensic services. The negative effects of being a speciality can also be addressed by thinking creatively about setting up rotational posts with other employers, whether at a basic grade or senior level. Given the competitive nature of the marketplace, consideration should be given to allowances and other conditions of service, including annual leave.

Stage 7 – Spreading the word

Spreading the word is both a process and an outcome combined. Given the geographical spread of therapists working in this field, significant challenges have to be surmounted in the gathering and disseminating of evidence and the sharing of experiences. However, we no longer have to rely only on face-to-face discussions and the odd few who get around to writing in journals to discuss their findings. Technology now offers us a plethora of opportunities to link up and carry out joint working in a way as never before. Therapists and other healthcare professionals are able to access research-funding opportunities with relative ease, but to date how many have done so?

Goodstein and Burke (1993 p.172), when discussing British Airways' success in change management, comment that 'the biggest problem now is in not so much to manage further change as it is to manage the change that has already occurred ... Managing momentum may be more difficult than managing change'. In other words, they (British Airways) have achieved significant change and success; now they must maintain what has been achieved while concentrating on continuing to be adaptable to changes in their external environment. This emphasizes the need for forensic occupational therapists to recognize the impact the profession has already made in working with mentally disordered offenders, but, in so doing, we must continue to move forward.

Conclusion

This chapter shares some of the key stages that occurred in setting up a successfully integrated occupational therapy service at the State Hospital. Important elements have included acquiring skills to assist the nursing team with the management of aggression. Working in high security, the occupational therapists have also had to learn to become risk managers. Initially, we began by focusing occupational therapy intervention where it was thought core professional skills would be most effective, that is with patients who have severe and enduring, treatment-resistant mental illness and those with challenging behaviour. Intervention may be ward based or undertaken in the occupational therapy department. Wherever it takes place, a constant endeavour is to ensure the activity meets the individual's and not the organization's needs. Using the principles of good communication, coordination, planning and collaboration should assist therapists in effectively spreading the word that the challenges and rewards of working in this field are great indeed. With evaluation and research, the profession is now ready to take its next step to advanced practice in this area.

References

College of Occupational Therapists (2000) Baroness Dean: Reduce shortage in three years. Occupational Therapy News 8(3) 1.

College of Occupational Therapists (2001) Standards of Practice for Occupational Therapists Working in Forensic Residential Settings. London: College of Occupational Therapists.

Department of Health (2000) Meeting the Challenge: A Strategy for the Allied Health Professions. London: Department of Health.

Duncan E (1999) Forensic services and occupational therapy: A developing area of practice? Occupational Therapy News 7(10) 24.

Goffman E (1961) Asylums: Essays on the Social Situations of Mental Patients and Other Inmates. Harmondsworth: Penguin Books.

Goodstein L and Burke W (1993) Creating successful organisation change. In: Managing Change (2nd edition), Mabey C and Mayon-White B (eds.). London: Paul Chapman Publishing Ltd.

Kielhofner G (1997) The Conceptual Foundations of Occupational Therapy (2nd edition). Philadelphia: F. A. Davis Company.

Lloyd C (1987) Forensic Psychiatry for Healthcare Professionals. Edinburgh: Chapman Hall.

Ritchie J, Dick D and Lingham R (1994) Report of the Inquiry into the Care and Treatment of Christopher Clunis. London: HMSO.

Scottish Health Advisory Service (1990) Report of Visit to the State Hospital, 1–9 October. Edinburgh: Scottish Health Advisory Service.

CHAPTER 13

Security issues for occupational therapists working in a medium secure setting

ANDREA NEESON AND REBECCA KELLY

Introduction

Security is an intrinsic part of the treatment of mentally disordered offenders, not only to protect the individual but also to protect staff, other patients and the public. Staff working within a forensic setting must have access to relevant induction and training in all aspects of the management of aggression, to equip them with the skills they need. Clinical risk assessment is an important part of treatment planning throughout a patient's in-patient admission and in their discharge planning. In order to maximize the effectiveness of security measures, clinical risk assessment and the development of policies and procedures are the responsibility of the whole multidisciplinary team. These measures do become second nature when working within a forensic environment, and underpin all practice.

Risk assessment and management form a primary part of any psychiatric patient's plan of care. It is clearly a particular issue with the forensic patient group. There is an increased focus on risk assessment in forensic psychiatry following high-profile community incidents involving individuals with mental illness (Ryan 1996). Risk assessment should be seen as a global approach to address both clinical and non-clinical issues. Assessing the degree of risk relating to a specific individual is vital both during an in-patient period of care and in attempting to predict and minimize future offending on discharge. Non-clinical risk assessment addresses those aspects, particularly relating to the environment and to health and safety considerations.

The focus of this chapter is on clinical and non-clinical security issues relating to risk in the setting-up and running of an in-patient secure occupational therapy service. It addresses the needs of a medium secure population but ideas can be extended to both low and high secure settings. This chapter will review:

- security and conflict within the therapeutic relationship

- training requirements for staff
- personal safety
- physical security including policy development and environmental management
- clinical risk assessment.

Security and the therapeutic relationship

The engagement of the patient in their care is central to any effective treatment plan. It is unlikely that changes to an individual's beliefs, attitudes and behaviour can be made unless the therapist and the patient have agreed goals and have developed a relationship in which trust is a central factor. In many mental health settings, patients have some degree of autonomy and choice about their treatment. However, in forensic settings, consideration is given to the impact of the individual's offending behaviour on society, and this is often in conflict with the patient's own beliefs about their risk. Patients will often hold the belief that they were mentally ill at the time of committing their offence and therefore when the mental illness is treated they no longer need detention or pose any form of risk. Others may not see fully the impact their offence has had on their family, or on the community, and feel that individuals should be more understanding towards them owing to their having a mental illness. Not only are patients subject to detention but they have also been assessed as requiring an environment that can offer some containment and control.

Personal experience suggests that many patients will express the belief that they are inappropriately detained and do not require conditions of security. It is rare, particularly early in their admission, that patients have sufficient insight to recognize they present a risk. Consequently, it is common to find that patients actively resist attempts to engage them in any therapeutic alliance and will fight against what they see as an unfair system. It is common for patients to use avoidance techniques such as staying in bed, arranging other appointments or complaining of physical symptoms to avoid engaging in treatment.

Staff must be very aware of the 'us and them' syndrome, in the knowledge that the balance of power does lie with the multidisciplinary team. Patients often feel that they cannot trust staff or they view staff as the people who hold the keys that keep them 'locked away'. Goffman (1961) argues that nurses and patients often view the climate within a secure ward very differently. Nurses may feel they are placing an emphasis on psychiatric care in a therapeutic environment by using interventions such as privilege systems, restraint, seclusion and medication. However, patients perceive these interventions to be humiliating punishment or forced containment. Occupational therapists are in the fortunate position of not usually being the ones who have to impose boundaries or procedures on the patients such as limits on leave from the unit, medication and access to personal belongings. Nurses are usually the ones placed in the difficult position of carrying through decisions made by the clinical team. This is an important issue for occupational therapists to be aware of. They need both to support their colleagues and to avoid splitting mechanisms. For example, a patient within our service approached an occupational therapist on a Monday morning and requested that she arrange community leave for him. The patient was aware that because of an incident at the weekend he had no community leave until he had been reviewed in the clinical team meeting. He went to the occupational therapist knowing that she had not been working at the weekend and may not have been aware of the decision made following the incident. This example also highlights the importance of receiving a full handover after any time away from the ward.

When patients are admitted, particularly if they have not encountered conditions of security before, the experience can be frightening. One patient, who had never previously been in a secure environment, found it so frightening and intimidating that he became more withdrawn on admission and spent most of his time isolating himself in his room. Patients are often traumatized by what has happened and are very unclear about what is expected of them. Understanding this subjective experience, and accurately reflecting this understanding, through empathy, during the initial assessment, is vital to the future of the therapeutic alliance. Patients need to feel that they can trust their carers and experience safety and containment within their environment.

Other patients will have experienced conditions of security often within a prison setting. This can strongly influence their attitudes towards both the staff and the environment, and they may not understand the role of treatment. It is not uncommon for patients to attempt to apply the unwritten rules established within the prison system to the hospital environment, such as attaching a hierarchy to offences and having an unwritten rule that patients will not 'snitch on each other'. The language associated with prison life is commonly used and words such as 'screws', 'parole' and 'doing time' can pervade the community. Again, this can be detrimental to the therapeutic relationship, as patients are looking toward release rather than engagement. It is therefore vital to have a thorough understanding of a patient's history, to know their background and adjust the way you approach the patients about engaging in their treatment.

'Occupational performance is influenced by the environmental context and content which may enhance or impede learning and performance' (Hagedorn 1997 p.122). The development of psychosocial skills, which for many patients is a key aspect of their treatment, needs to be transferable where feasible to different environmental settings. It is clear that a secure environment is inconsistent with personal autonomy and the development of an internal locus of control. Many decisions are taken on behalf of the patient. It is part of the occupational therapist's role to attempt to minimize outward signs of security and seek ways to empower patients within the context of their environment. Hendry (1993) (cited in Tarbuck et al. 1999) states that there should be more emphasis placed on therapeutic participation rather than on matters of security. There are a number of ways this can be done, for example allowing patients to have an element of choice over their occupational therapy programme or showing patients that you are giving them responsibility by trusting them to use sharp tools safely. Another way is to minimize the visual signs of security. Examples include: having any tools out before the sessions so that patients do not see the signing-in and -out procedure, having slam-lock doors (so that staff are not seen to be locking doors all of the time) and keeping keys on a belt on a discreet retractable key fob rather than hanging down on a chain.

Training requirements for staff

Staff must always be aware of the safety of the patients, themselves and their colleagues. Often these skills are developed through experience and knowledge, but there is no substitute for good supervision and targeted training.

Management of aggression

The presence of mental illness, personality disorder and, on occasion, substance misuse, together with a tendency towards impulsive behaviour, can produce a volatile mixture. The best way to manage violence is to prevent it. Sometimes even the knowledge that a patient is unpredictable can help staff to devise a management plan. Particular skills are needed to deal with aggressive behaviour. Specifically these include self-awareness, understanding of the impact of verbal and non-verbal behaviour within interactions, and use of other de-escalation techniques. Attention to the environment can decrease the likelihood of violence. A quiet ward, individual rooms, ward routine, group meetings, staff accessibility and clear expectations of acceptable behaviour all help to frame a safe environment.

Breakaway techniques

Breakaway techniques, like control and restraint, should be part of the induction process for all staff, including occupational therapists. Again, it is something that no staff member would wish to have to use, and yet it is vital to be equipped with the skills to escape a situation safely if necessary. Breakaway techniques involve the minimal possible use of force to enable an individual to escape from a range of attacks against them. It is essential training for those who have to work alone and who may be at risk from the patient because of the nature of their work.

Control and restraint

Control and restraint is the main practical training available for the last resort management of violence. The course offers comprehensive training for the management of patients in care settings who exhibit violent behaviour. The techniques are aimed at maximizing the safety of all concerned. The aim is to control the situation, prevent the individual from causing further harm and give the team the option to deal with the situation quietly and quickly by moving the patient to another suitable room or location. Clearly, physical restraint should be avoided wherever possible. Verbal de-escalation techniques in most cases will be successful; however, it is pointless and potentially dangerous *to hope* that these techniques will succeed on every occasion.

Within our service, control and restraint training is integral to the induction programme for occupational therapists. Narrative accounts and experience suggest that serious incidents occur very rarely within an activity environment. An audit was carried out at the Oxford Clinic that looked at the number of reported incidents over a period of 13 months (Garman 2000). It showed there were 137 incidents involving physical restraint, three of which were in the sports hall; the rest took place on the ward. There were no incidents in the activity area. Nevertheless, even one serious incident is too many. All staff need to be prepared to deal with these eventualities.

Our service places a high priority on close team working and consequently the occupational therapist spends considerable amounts of time on the ward. It is our belief that there is no advantage to expect the nursing team to be the ones solely responsible for containing violence, nor does it enhance good team working. There are occasions when there may be small numbers of nursing staff on duty and the occupational therapist is required to assist in managing incidents. Commonly, the occupational therapist, if not required as part of the control and restraint team, can still offer support by calming other patients distressed by the incident and minimizing disruption to the ward.

The conflict between the potential for damage to the therapeutic relationship and the critical need for effective team working will always be an issue. Our experience tends to show that patients forget incidents in which they have been restrained and in which staff members were involved. One female patient who was restrained by a team including an occupational therapist showed no hostility or anger towards any of the team and continued to engage in her occupational therapy programme as soon as it was believed to be appropriate.

Search

There will be occasions within any forensic setting that patients will attempt to obtain banned or illegal contraband items or substances. Occupational therapists should be particularly aware that workshop areas not only hold many potentially dangerous items such as woodwork tools but also provide a good hiding area because of the amount of equipment and materials being stored. These are also areas that tend not to be searched as frequently as the wards and are accessible to most of the patients within the unit.

Developing the skill of searching is as much a responsibility for occupational therapists as it is for other members of the team. The occupational therapy service needs to demonstrate responsibility and accountability for areas they manage. Our service has engaged in specialized training with the police force in search techniques. This training is now cascading down to all staff, and the occupational therapy service has been active in involving itself in this process.

Relevant legislation

1. Occupational therapists need working knowledge of the Mental Health Act (1983) – specifically those sections relating to Home Office restrictions and prison orders. These have significant impact on the individual's occupational therapy programme, owing to restrictions on community leave and the need to coordinate and agree care packages with the Home Office. For some patients, discharge into the community is not an option, as they will be returning to the prison system to complete a sentence. It is very important that occupational therapists are aware of the implications of the different types of detention, as this will guide the treatment aims and outcome. Forensic occupational therapists, like other occupational therapists working in mental health, are subject to all other Mental Health Act (1983) requirements including, but not exclusively, Section 17 and second opinion for consent to treatment. The reforms to the Mental Health Act (Department of Health 2000) set out a strategy to improve mental health services in England and intend to be fully compatible with the new Human Rights Act (1998). The new reforms propose the inclusion of a wider definition of the term 'mental disorder' which includes high risk, personality disordered patients, to ensure they receive good quality services with a greater emphasis on therapeutic treatment (Ling Boey and Sealey-Lapes 2001).

2. The Human Rights Act (1998) recognizes that all individuals have certain minimal and fundamental human rights, for example the right to a fair trial and fair hearing and the right to life. If a human right is breached, a client will be able to take their complaint to a court or tribunal in the UK. There are articles within the Human Rights Act (1998) that all professionals need to be aware of and consider when working with patients in conditions of security. For example, Article 5 relates to liberty and security, and Article 6 to rights to a fair trial.
3. All employees should be aware of their rights and responsibilities under the Health and Safety at Work Act (1974). For those working in secure environments, there is a section relating to risk assessment and violence, stating that it is the agency's duty to ensure employees' safety against violence and aggression as far as possible.

Personal safety

Apart from the training requirements described above, there are a number of other measures to be taken to ensure personal safety. These include:

Confidentiality

It is always important to maintain a professional relationship with patients. In forensic services, many of the patients will present with personality disorder as a primary diagnosis or in addition to mental illness. One of the problems associated with people who have a personality disorder is dysfunctional interpersonal relationships, and it is not uncommon for patients to use information about staff inappropriately. Any personal information relating to one's self or colleagues, given to a patient, is potentially dangerous and should always be avoided. There are ways to distract from and avoid answering questions of this sort, for example referring the question back to the patient and asking why they want to know that information. Alternatively, it can be explained why you do not feel it is appropriate to be answering, or stating firmly that you are not going to answer such questions. Where a good rapport with the patient has been developed, humour may be a useful way to move on to a different subject.

Boundary setting

Clear messages and consistency in approach will avoid some of the problems associated with boundary testing. Patients will often 'test' how far their inappropriate behaviour will be tolerated. Setting clear boundaries is much more effective if there is consistency in approach amongst the staff group. This is particularly evident with patients diagnosed with borderline personality disorder, who may develop emotionally unstable and intense personal relationships usually with particular members of staff. These patients may become very dependent on certain members of staff and will often insist on talking to that individual when they are feeling distressed. This not only places a lot of pressure on individual members of staff but also allows the patient to split staff groups and manipulate staff members.

Physical surroundings

Awareness of one's physical position should always be considered, particularly when working alone with a patient. Common sense dictates that it is sensible to place oneself near a door and to be aware of potential escape routes. Familiarization with emergency resources such as wall alarms or personal alarms should form part of all staff induction programmes. These issues become second nature with experience; however, therapists should be aware of not compromising the therapeutic relationship because of these concerns. Examples include setting up a room before a session so that it is not obvious to a patient that you are setting up a room considering your escape route or encouraging escorts to participate in a group as much as possible and not to stand watching over patients. It is also essential to let other staff know your location, who you are working with, any escort requirements you may need and the appropriateness of using potentially dangerous items during sessions.

Non-verbal cues

Non-verbal cues are often the most accessible information about how a person is feeling. Tense, upright postures can indicate anxiety or anger, and these can be easily picked up. Patients need to feel safe and confident, and there is nothing less reassuring than a nervous/timid therapist. Sitting down and looking interested, with a relaxed posture, can help defuse tense situations.

Policy development and environmental management

This section will deal specifically with safety issues relating to the areas where occupational therapists offer much of their treatment such as workshops, sports facilities and kitchens. These areas commonly hold equipment that can be classed as 'sharps'. That is they have the potential to be used as dangerous weapons or instruments for self-injury and hence must be carefully monitored. In our experience, safety issues should be clarified and agreed upon before allowing patient access. One way of achieving this is the development of detailed policies and procedures for each area, providing clear guidance to all staff. These should be read and understood before staff are allowed access to or given responsibility for these areas.

Policies provide general statements on the organization and running of a service. Procedures are more specific guides, putting policies into practice. In general, policies should include a consideration of the following:

- a description of the service and resources available
- overall responsibility for management and coordination
- types of activities to be conducted
- types of patients expected to access the facility
- supervision of the area, including minimum escort numbers
- referral procedures and risk assessment
- team coordination and the movement of patients
- action in the event of emergency
- management of sharps
- management of substances hazardous to health (e.g. adhesives, paints, solvents)
- use of technical equipment such as lathes, kilns, computer technology, etc.
- review date of policy

All policies need to be understood and adhered to by staff if they are going to be effective. Therefore, the team should have the opportunity to read and agree any policies in draft form and make comments to allow for amendment before implementation. All services are subject to change; incorporating a review date will allow for changes in practice and promote flexibility. All policies and procedures should be immediately accessible to staff and form part of the induction process.

There are a number of areas in which the occupational therapist provides treatment and security procedures and considerations for these are shown in Table 13.1. Security will be addressed within other general policies such as sharps, escorts, medical emergency, hostage-taking and fire drills. These policies are unit wide and applied to all staff to promote consistency. Specific procedures should be available and assigned to each policy area. In our experience, having some procedures to guide practice has minimized potential conflict and confusion and ensured the safe management of activity areas. Other areas to consider which may benefit from procedural guidance include sports facilities, garden areas, kitchen and community facilities.

Table 13.1 Security procedures and considerations

Area	Procedural Considerations
Information Technology	• Password protection • Access to passwords • Monitoring of use • Vetting of software • Minimum computing knowledge for supervising staff • Storage of patient work, for example using floppy disk or hard drive • Preparation of area • IT support • Use of computing for clinical purposes and confidentiality issues • Use of printer and monitoring work content removed from area • Internet access • Out-of-hours use • Monitoring of materials and equipment and budgetary constraints
Workshop	• Clinical risk assessment prior to individual patients access • Coordination of areas • Maximum numbers of patients • Minimum number of escorts • Emergency procedures – including evacuation, fire noticeboards, hostage-taking and medical emergency • Identification of key coordinator for these procedures • Health and safety issues such as COSHH, use of aprons, dust masks, other protective clothing, etc. • Communication with wards • Out-of-hours use • Required qualifications for use of technical equipment
Safe Keeping of Sharps	• Locking sharp utensils in cupboards • Listing all sharps • Weekly checks and recording • Signing-out procedures prior to sessions • Accounting procedures post-session • Allocating responsibilities for sharps to named staff • Monitoring the sharps during sessions • Procedures in case of items going missing, including initiating search procedures

Clinical risk assessment and management

Ryan (1996) suggests that clinical risk assessment is about predicting the future and the likelihood of particular events occurring. It involves gathering information about certain aspects of the patient's history and behaviour, such as history of violence, self-harm, mental illness, compliance and insight. Two published tools that are designed for assessing risk are *Violent Offenders – Appraising and Managing Risk* (Vernon et al. 1998) and the *HCR-20 Assessing Risk for Violence* (Webster et al. 1997). The importance of risk assessment in forensic psychiatry is widely accepted; however, it has little meaning unless practical measures to manage risks can be implemented following the assessment. Prior to any patient being allowed into an area which may provide access to potential weapons, a consideration of the risk to themselves and others must be made. This consideration should be documented and reflect the team's discussion and agreement. There needs to be a built-in mechanism for review, and the risk assessment should be accessible.

Different services are likely to have their own process for risk assessment. Sometimes it will form part of a clinical team meeting or ward round and sometimes a more formal mechanism may be used such as a referral form. Whichever is felt to be the most appropriate method, documentation is essential to demonstrate that risks have been fully considered. The College of Occupational Therapists has published standard guidelines for secure settings which specify the need to record risk in occupational therapy notes (College of Occupational Therapists 2001). It is suggested that some agreed format be implemented for consistency and quality control. The areas that need to be considered include:

- leave status/observation level
- legal detention status
- historical and fixed risk factors including previous offending history, use of weapons, history of suicide attempt and self-harm, drug and alcohol abuse, psychopathic traits (including personality disorder assessments, etc.)
- dynamic risk factors including mental state, stressors, relationship issues, changeable factors known to influence behaviour
- other factors to consider include compliance with treatment, degree of insight, impulsiveness and current risk to self
- environmental – specific access agreements to areas, for example access to computing but not woodwork, etc.
- keyworker details
- timetable.

The types of information needed on any risk assessment pro forma will depend on the way the occupational therapy service relates to the team. In some cases the occupational therapist will be very closely linked to the ward and may operate a blanket referral system; in other cases they may accept only individual referrals.

Conclusion

It is hoped that this chapter has given the reader some understanding of security issues when working in conditions of medium security. The examples given are based on a medium secure setting, although the information is transferable to conditions of low and high security. The chapter has highlighted professional issues for therapists such as training requirements and boundary setting as well as practical issues such as policy development that can be adopted within a service. The chapter has emphasized the need for a team approach when carrying out risk assessments as well as recommending the implementation of practical measures to manage risk. It is hoped that the security measures discussed within this chapter are adopted and underpin the practice of all staff working within a secure environment.

References

Boey ML and Sealey-Lapes C (2001) Reforming the Mental Health Act: What does it mean for occupational therapists? Occupational Therapy News 9(2):10.

College of Occupational Therapists (2002) The Standards for Practice: Occupational Therapy in Forensic Residential Settings. London: College of Occupational Therapists.

Department of Health (2000) Reforming the Mental Health Act, Summary. London: The Stationery Office.

Garman G (2000) Reported Incidents at the Oxford Clinic. A 13-month study of incidents (unpublished).

Goffman E (1961) Asylums: Essays on the Social Situation of Inpatients and Other Inmates. Harmondsworth: Penguin.

Hagedorn R (1997) Foundations for Practice in Occupational Therapy (2nd edition). Edinburgh: Churchill Livingstone.

Health and Safety at Work Act (1974) London: HMSO.

Human Rights Act (1998) London: HMSO.

Mental Health Act (1983) London: HMSO.

Ryan T (1996) Risk management and people with mental health problems. In: Good Practice in Risk Assessment and Risk Management 1, Kemshall H and Pritchard J (eds.). London: Jessica Kingsley Publishers.

Tarbuck P, Topping Morris B and Burnard P (1999) Forensic Mental Health Nursing. Strategy and Implementation. London: Whurr.

Vernon L, Quinsey V, Harris G, Rice M and Cormier C (1998) Violent Offenders – Appraising and Managing Risk. Washington DC: American Psychological Association.

Webster C, Douglas K, Eaves D and Hart S (1997) HCR-20 Assessing Risk for Violence, Version 2. Vancouver: Mental Health Law, and Policy Institute, Simon Fraser University.

CHAPTER 14

Team working and liaison

HELENA HOLFORD AND DEBORAH ALRED

Introduction

> Psychiatry involves the difficult task of disentangling symptoms and illness-
> es which are not just physical. They routinely involve damaging past expe-
> riences, stressful situations, family problems or the use of drugs or alcohol,
> as well as more medical problems. So it is realistic to take as broad a view
> as possible of the things that might be producing any individual patient's
> problems. That's why we need people from different backgrounds, with
> different trainings, different skills and different ways of approaching
> problems.   (Royal College of Psychiatrists 2002)

However, a range of professionals in itself is not sufficient. These
people must be able to work together in an integrated and cooperative
manner. Good team working is fundamental to the quality of forensic
services. This chapter aims to communicate its importance and value to
the work of the forensic occupational therapist. Team working for forensic occupational therapists can be one of the sources of greatest job
satisfaction – and greatest frustration. In this chapter we consider how
current trends and legislation are aimed at supporting integrated team
working. Sometimes the professional behaviours that support, or diminish, team working occur in the tacit domain, that is they are often not
spoken about, articulated or discussed. The expertise of other authors is
used to identify key elements that foster positive teamwork. We also draw
on our personal experience of working in medium secure settings to
highlight issues and to outline simple strategies that enhance good liaison
and team working. The chapter begins with a look at language and considers the intricacy of defining multidisciplinary team working.

The language of teams

Just defining 'team' can be problematic. For there are groups of professionals who work toward a common goal but who may not identify

themselves as working in a multidisciplinary team. There are also groups of health and social care professionals, designated as a team, who experience fundamental problems stemming from the relationships between them.

And who is in the team? Do we include the patient's individual care team? Or perhaps it is the ward-environment team. Or is it the wider health and social care team? And is the patient part of the team? In the smaller secure forensic settings, identifying the team may be easier than in the larger units and special hospitals, or in a community setting. For practitioners reading this book, wherever you are based, it may be worth considering who is in your team.

Additionally, 'different professionals in the same team can have dissimilar and conflicting understandings of the nature of "effective teamwork"' (Miller et al. 2001 p.2). Does working together include the tasks of professional practice or decision-making too? If decision-making is included, it is interesting to consider whether equal weight is given to the contribution of all team members.

The terms multiprofessional, multidisciplinary, interdisciplinary and interprofessional are sometimes used synonymously. Mandy (1996) in clarifying multidisciplinary and interdisciplinary describes 'multidisciplinary' as a team where everyone works in parallel. Each discipline is required to do his, or her, own thing with little or no awareness of others' work. On the other hand, he says successful interdisciplinary teams demonstrate the following characteristics:

- goal directedness, where the team has a central purpose, providing a rationale for its establishment
- disciplinary articulation, which requires understanding from all members of each other's role and recognizing areas of overlap
- communication, appreciating how others understand knowledge, how this is gained and used
- flexibility, which includes essential attributes such as open-mindedness, tolerance and valuing of different perspectives, acceptance in changes in authority and the desire for challenge
- conflict resolution, seen as the ability to overcome difficulties and conflict.

An extensive research study into how well different health and social care professionals work together reveals fascinating and complex patterns of clinical team working (Miller et al. 2001). In this study, whole multiprofessional teams were observed in action. The research identified and named three types of multiprofessional working: 'integrated', 'fragmented' and 'core and periphery'.

The **integrated collaborative** team is described as existing in an organizational context of stability. Team members were not called away to contribute to other teams; this allowed team allegiance and identity to develop. Fundamental to this type of team working was openness in communication. Commitment to joint practices and good communication established a strong and safe learning environment. This was 'manifested by a high level of understanding about individual contributions to patient care, and knowledge about where specific roles met or overlapped' (Miller 2001 p.32).

Fragmented team working led to patient management – including problem-solving, decision-making and responsibilities for action – falling to single professional groups. Communication was relatively brief and related more to the giving of information than to the sharing of professional perspectives or clinical reasoning. Role understanding was superficial, with members unable or unwilling to develop in-depth understanding of others' roles. In this context, many professionals actively protected their role boundaries (Miller et al. 2001).

In the **core and periphery** teams, there was an integrated multiprofessional core, the remainder of the team being peripheral to that core. This delineation was not caused by the role the professional undertook in the patients' care. On the contrary 'it related to those who could and possibly should have been closely collaborating with other members of the team' (Miller et al. 2001 p.41). Within the core, many integrated practices existed such as multiprofessional assessment and communication systems that encouraged in-depth discussion. But this positive working did not extend to those on the periphery. Communication between core and periphery was constrained, and there was a lack of understanding of how the roles of people in the periphery come together with those in the core to provide more comprehensive care.

The benefits of integrated, collaborative working included continuity, consistency, a reduced number of ambiguous messages, actions resulting from a holistic perspective and improved problem-solving. Detrimental outcomes were noted for both other types of team working. We suspect all forensic teams aspire to achieve an integrated, collaborative model of team working, but we leave it to the practitioners reading this book to decide which kind of team they are presently working in. In the meantime, 'multidisciplinary team' will be the term used here.

Occupational therapy in the forensic multidisciplinary team

For occupational therapists working within forensic services, a number of factors highlight the need for good team working and liaison. First, there are the needs of the clients, which are complex and challenging. Their

needs can be met only by the pooled expertise of a range of professionals carefully coordinated with each other. Second, the intensive staffing
levels within a secure unit mean that, in practice, the team the occupational therapist will be liaising and working with may be very large. Shift
patterns and night duty often result in unpredictable staff rosters, which
can affect the continuity of communication. Third, occupational therapy
is often carried out within the wards, the therapy environment being
more physically closely integrated within the unit than in other speciali-
ties. This means that the effectiveness of occupational therapists relies on
multidisciplinary cooperation and understanding. Thus, communication
needs to involve close, day-to-day monitoring and feedback as well as
adherence to an agreed overall plan. The consequences for not working
closely within a multidisciplinary framework can put the occupational
therapist, other disciplines and residents at risk with this potentially dangerous client group.

In a medium secure setting at any one time occupational therapists can
perceive themselves as being in several teams: the occupational therapy
team, the ward team consisting primarily of occupational therapists and
nurses, and the wider multidisciplinary team. The combination of all
these factors means that occupational therapists must put a great deal of
concentrated, systematic effort into both formal and informal communication in order to function effectively within the multidisciplinary
framework.

Current trends and legislation

Since 1975, in health and social care generally, 'Governments have
endorsed collaborative working, both between different disciplines and
different agencies. More recently there has developed an over-riding conviction that working in partnership is essential in order to realise the
good-quality, effective services to which the Government aspires'
(Norman et al. 1998 p.3). This is echoed in the latest Government initiatives, including the NHS Plan which emphasizes the importance of
multidisciplinary working and flexibility in the use of skill development,
the focus being on the patient at the centre of the planning and treatment
process (Department of Health 2000a). The NHS Plan stresses the importance of developing care protocols, identifying how common conditions
should be managed, and which staff should be involved. It is expected
that allied health professionals will benefit greatly from this protocol-
based approach (Department of Health 2000b).

Likewise, the Care Programme Approach (CPA) (Department of Health
1999) addresses team working and liaison. The patient-focused, holistic
approach of the CPA fits in well with occupational therapy philosophy.

Increasingly, the coordination of the occupational therapy role within the team is being facilitated through this approach, which has the following essential elements:

- systematic arrangements for assessing the health and social needs of people accepted into specialist mental health services
- the formulation of a care plan which identifies the health and social care required from a variety of providers
- the appointment of a care coordinator to keep in close touch with the service user and to monitor and coordinate care
- regular review and, where necessary, agreement to changes to the care plans.

Within a forensic unit the most likely format is a three- to six-monthly CPA review where each discipline compiles a report monitoring the patient's past and present progress and setting recommendations and an action plan for the future. The coordination of the action plan allows the occupational therapist to identify what would be appropriate for their role and what activities are necessary, but which another team member could carry out.

The importance of a coordinated and complementary use of different professional skills to meet the needs of the client group is increasingly being recognized in this legislation and in current planning trends. Work on competency-based frameworks has been conducted by the National Board for Scotland (2001) and the Sainsbury Centre for Mental Health (2001). This work identifies specific specialist competencies for working in forensic services. Specific forensic competencies are seen as above and beyond basic training for all professions and as shared skills that can be developed in joint training. This concept leads the way for shared-skills development, learned in the workplace, which also has the potential to enhance the multidisciplinary culture.

Similarly, joint training in generic, treatment-specific skills can ensure the service provides a broad spectrum of treatment approaches. The National Board for Scotland (2001) identified the following examples:

- cognitive behaviour therapy
- psychosocial interventions
- psychodynamic therapy
- anger management
- dialectical behaviour therapy
- offence-specific approaches
- treatment to address substance abuse.

In a medium secure setting the occupational therapist can also use their profession-specific skills to facilitate joint working, particularly when training and encouraging staff in activity and group planning and development. Occupational therapists have a duty to balance their time between more generic responsibilities and continuing to provide a specific occupational therapy service. This need for balance, to promote positive team working, can also be seen in the chapter 'Setting up a forensic occupational therapy service' in this book.

The experience of team working in a medium secure environment

So what is it like working as a forensic occupational therapist? In this speciality, more perhaps than any other, it is essential to give sufficient time for communication. Spending time with individual staff, sharing professional perspectives by explaining what you are trying to achieve and becoming aware of their priorities are absolute requirements of practice. Involvement and inclusion of staff will pay dividends. Because of the size of the team, it is important to expect to spend correspondingly more time on communication. There is little published evidence about working in a multidisciplinary team on a forensic unit; however, the experience of multidisciplinary teams in other areas helps to deepen understanding. For example, Øvretveit (1995) suggests a multidisciplinary team without conflict is a contradiction in terms. He says that the point of a team is to bring together the different skills that a patient needs and to combine them in a way that is not possible outside a team. He emphasizes that problems in reaching or carrying out collective decisions in teams are rarely due to 'personality clashes' alone. They are often because an individual's responsibilities, or accountability, prevent them from agreeing or reaching collective decisions. This tension can lead to professions staying within their uni-professional cultures. It is all too easy for the shared objective to be lost and each separate profession to work alongside each other rather than with each other. This creates a situation where confusions and conflict can occur between the professions.

One strategy that can enhance positive multidisciplinary working is having a shared vision. In their study, Miller et al. (2001) observe that the integrated, collaborative team had largely developed a shared philosophy of care. This provided the basis for joint-working practices. 'This approach aimed to secure the optimum quality of patient rehabilitation, rather than simply functional improvement' (Miller et al. 2001 p.34). Grappling with and developing a core, articulated philosophy, which is congruent with the various different disciplines' beliefs, can promote good team working. Each profession must draw on its own theories, but some units are able to encompass these in 'a strong clear philosophy or working style' (Fairbairn 2000 p.293). This principle is developed further in the chapter 'The foundation of good practice' in Part One of this book.

Collaboration, which is so essential for good team working, flourishes only in an atmosphere where there is a high level of trust among disciplines (Akhavin et al. 1999). Team members can assume accountability and responsibility for patient care more easily where trust and respect for individual professional perspectives are part of the team culture. Øvretveit (1995) suggests that a way for a working team culture to develop is through clear team decision-making protocols and time being made for open discussion when issues arise.

For example, one scenario common to forensic occupational therapists involves risk assessment and discussion about whether individual patients can participate in certain activities. If the clinical reasoning that underpins the choice of activity is not understood by the team, these interventions can be perceived merely as treats or rewards. Some team members may feel the patient is receiving preferential treatment inappropriate to his or her behaviour on the ward, rather than recognizing that the activity is designed to meet identified needs. An example of this kind of conflict can be seen in the case of Gary.

Case example

Gary is detained under Sections 37/41 of the Mental Health Act for actual bodily harm. He has episodes of very aggressive behaviour, and he finds the closed environment of a secure setting difficult to cope with. He suffers from paranoid schizophrenia. However, he has settled periods where he attends occupational therapy sessions regularly and progresses well. As a result of his general improvement, he gained Home Office escorted community leave for four hours per week. He then displayed a series of aggressive outbursts, one towards a staff member and two towards other clients. The reason behind these outbursts would appear to be his anxiety about entering the community after two years in a secure setting. Consequently, the team stopped Gary's leave. Gary again settled and was rewarded with the reinstatement of his Home Office leave.

Careful risk assessment will need to be carried out by the staff involved in Gary's care. Planning and discussion at this stage will limit the chance of disagreement if Gary's leave is stopped. This communication is two-way. It is important for the occupational therapist to explain the rationale behind each trip and its relevance to the overall assessment and treatment package. It is also important for the nursing staff to describe Gary's behaviour on the unit, including his interactions with other residents and how the staff interpret his mental state. From this foundation, a realistic joint plan for the community trips can be devised, possibly with both nursing and occupational therapy staff acting as escorts. In a busy medium secure unit these discussions and intensive planning with written records take time but are vital. Yet, despite good forward planning, problems can arise on the day of the trip. It is possible for a different group of ward staff, who have not been party to the shared clinical reasoning, to be on duty at the time of the trip and cancel it at the last minute. This is where a clear written protocol, outlining the thinking behind the trip, can ensure an appropriate decision is made.

One study into multidisciplinary team working asked seven different disciplines to consider interprofessional working in adult community mental health teams (Norman et al. 1998). First, each uni-professional group was asked to formulate a consensual account of their own professional identities, roles and responsibilities. Then they had to identify the issues that arose for their own profession in respect of the roles and responsibilities of each of the other professions. The occupational therapists' story illustrated that occupational therapists generally feel positive about their professional identity but feel misunderstood and undervalued by other mental healthcare professionals. In fact, the other professional groups valued the occupational therapists' skills and approach to patients, but they also called for clarification of the role. It is clear that occupational therapists need to develop and improve the way they put across occupational therapy to other disciplines.

Occupational therapists often find themselves explaining what they do. In an in-patient setting this is essential for effective interventions; however, some may want to think about giving a more detailed account of their clinical reasoning. For example, if the occupational therapist plans a quiz, the questions will be selected according to the skills, interests and specialist knowledge of the participants. The quiz may be structured around meeting the identified needs of some of the individuals in the group. For example, using teams and scoring on a board to promote cooperation and awareness of others, or giving individuals answer sheets in order for them to work at their own pace. Ward staff will have a role in reassuring and encouraging residents to participate. They will need to strike a balance between participating, and so providing an example to residents, and not taking over and answering all the questions, thereby potentially undermining residents' confidence in themselves. The occupational therapist will need to ensure that this supportive role is understood if the session is going to be a success.

Structures for communication

Collaboration and good communication, so essential for positive team working, can frequently be enhanced through quite simple and practical measures. Some of these were identified in a study of psychiatric rehabilitation units by Fairburn (2000) and work just as well in forensic units.

Meetings

There are a number of multidisciplinary meetings held on the unit providing forums for clear communication and the development of an integrated team approach. Ward rounds, case conferences and care programme reviews all offer time to focus on specific issues of resident care. An occupational therapist does need to be present at these, or if unable to be present at least to provide a brief, written report. Where good communication networks are still being established, it can be helpful to think through ahead of time the patient's participation in occupational therapy. Brief notes can then be taken to the meeting so that the essential aspects of clinical reasoning can be outlined. It is also useful to check how the oral contribution given to the meeting has been recorded. Our experience indicates that it is also important that handovers are attended by the occupational therapist. They are primarily for nursing staff to hand over the care of their patients to the next nursing shift. However, they are also a time when the occupational therapist can learn about any ward issues and inform the rest of the staff of any alterations to the programme.

Shared patient notes

Shared, or joint, patient note-keeping arrangements promote communication by maintaining all relevant information about the individual in the same place. Since taking up this system, we have found it has an additional benefit, through the informal contact of spending time in the nursing station. This has included sharing information orally, which assists with the development of mutual understanding and professional relationships. People will more readily ask, 'So what do you actually do then?' in a ward office than in a more formal situation. A recommended response to this question is to find out which residents they work closely with and tailor your response to that resident. This makes an immediately relevant impact. Fairburn (2000) notes that the inclusion of a group attendance register was found to enhance nurses' interest in groups, especially if mostly therapists ran the groups.

Written communication

The communication book and ward diary are also useful tools that are used to ensure that other team members know what is happening and to assist in information exchange. It is not an infallible system. There are occasions when, despite their use, other team members remain confused about information or do not attach sufficient weight to the entry. One former colleague acknowledged and dealt with this problem by writing the diary and communication book entries in luminous coloured pens. This action gained the right attention and became a personal trademark.

Sharing tasks

Involving others in the activity programme not only enriches the programme by utilizing the skills of other disciplines but also promotes more shared understanding and cooperation. The chapter 'Programme planning' in Part Two of this book develops this theme. A potential hazard of profession-specific working is that occupational therapists can be seen to be offering 'nice' things. On the other hand, nursing staff, for example, have the role of enforcing security, ensuring compliance with medication and often have to carry out methods of restraint. Involving nursing staff in activities and occupational therapists in security, including control and restraint, helps to minimize these unhelpful perceptions. It also promotes a higher level of understanding about the individual contributions to patient care, and knowledge of where specific roles meet or overlap.

Systems and protocols

A recent development in our services has been the use of joint risk assessment when planning a new activity or a group trip. This encourages different disciplines to sit down and think through the implications of the chosen activity from all angles, anticipating any possible problems and solutions. This has developed confidence in the activity and each person's role in its implementation. Similarly, all procedures and protocols are more likely to be owned and implemented if jointly developed.

Multidisciplinary team supervision and education

Although, in our experience, tutorials about the role of occupational therapy do not pay dividends, joint training on topics of mutual interest can be beneficial. For example, a multidisciplinary study day on substance-misuse issues develops skills and knowledge for the individual; it also builds mutual respect and trust within the team. We find joint-supervision arrangements can also help team working. This can be achieved either by bringing outside facilitators in for multiprofessional group supervision, or for staff to receive individual supervision from more senior members of different professions. It is important to remember that issues of role identity and effectiveness within the team are common to all professions and not just to occupational therapy. Fairburn (2000) notes that occupational therapists may be left out of the larger nursing teams' working and support systems. Although it can take some time to overcome initial reluctance, being involved with general ward support can help the forensic occupational therapist to be viewed as part of the in-patient team.

Conclusion

Multidisciplinary team working is a profoundly important aspect of the role of the forensic occupational therapist. Being part of an integrated collaborative team is also one of the deepest satisfactions of working in forensic services. Good team working demands committed attention to positive strategies that deepen understanding about each discipline's different roles and responsibilities. Some of the tactics suggested here appear simple but that does not diminish their effectiveness. The effort is in carrying them out consistently over a period of time. This chapter has highlighted different patterns of clinical team working and suggested some strategies that we have found helpful in promoting dynamic and coordinated multidisciplinary working.

References

Akhavin P, Amaral D, Murphy M and Uehlinger K (1999) Collaborative practice: A nursing perspective of the psychiatric interdisciplinary treatment team. Holistic Nursing Practise 13(2) 1–11.

Department of Health (1999) Effective Care Co-ordination in Mental Health Services: Modernising the Care Programme Approach. London: Department of Health.

Department of Health (2000a) The NHS Plan: A Plan for Investment, a Plan for Reform. London: The Stationery Office.

Department of Health (2000b) A Health Service of all the Talents: Developing the NHS Workforce. London: The Stationery Office.

Fairburn C (2000) Psychiatric rehabilitation units: How can occupational therapists help them into the new millennium. British Journal of Occupational Therapy 63(6) 291–293.

Mandy P (1996) Interdisciplinary rather than multidisciplinary or generic practice. British Journal of Therapy and Rehabilitation 3(2) 110–112.

Miller C, Freeman M and Ross N (2001) Interprofessional Practice in Health and Social Care. London: Arnold.

National Board for Scotland (2001) Continuing Professional Development Portfolio – A Route to Enhanced Competence in Forensic Mental Health Nursing. Edinburgh: National Board for Nursing, Midwifery and Health Visiting for Scotland. Available from NHS Education for Scotland.

Norman I, Peck E and Richards H (1998) Inter-professional Working in Adult Community Mental Health Services: Setting a Positive Agenda. Executive summary prepared on behalf of the King's Fund/CMHSD Adult Community Mental Health Services' National Reference and Development Groups. London: King's College.

Øvretveit J (1995) Team decision-making. Journal of Interprofessional Care 9(1) 41–51

Royal College of Psychiatrists (2002) The Mental Health Team – Fact sheet from the Royal College of Psychiatrists, downloaded from www.rcpsych.ac.uk/info/factsheets/pfacteam.htm on 31/10/02.

Sainsbury Centre for Mental Health (2001) The Capable Practitioner: A Framework and List of the Practitioner Capabilities Required to Implement the National Service Framework for Mental Health. A report commissioned by the National Service Framework Workforce Action Team. London: Sainsbury Centre for Mental Health, available from www.scmh.org.uk

PART FIVE

CLINICAL ISSUES

CHAPTER 15

Women in secure environments

KATHRYN HARRIS

Introduction

The question that may be most pertinent to answer is: what is it that makes women in secure settings so different from men? There are, of course, a number of similarities. On the surface, it would seem that most are suffering from a mental illness. Many come from deprived social backgrounds and have a history of criminal offences. However, if we look more closely at the type of women admitted to secure settings, there are marked differences. In fact, research carried out in 1999 (Stafford 1999) by a voluntary support group, Women in Special Hospitals (WISH – a charitable organization set up to support women in secure hospitals), highlighted a number of differences that were felt to be significant when compared with men in the high secure settings in England. These differences are echoed for women in medium secure settings. Marked differences for women include: greater numbers with a history of sexual abuse, having no experience of employment, lower ages at admission, different reasons for admission, more are parents, more have associated problems of alcohol misuse, and patterns of diagnosis are not the same as for men.

This chapter focuses specifically on the needs of women in medium security and aims to highlight some of those needs and how occupational therapists can attempt to treat what has been labelled a difficult patient group. It is based on the experience of therapists working mainly within services with dedicated women's beds and not where completely separate women's services are provided.

Improving provision – historical perspective

The Home Office and Department of Health (1992) reviewed the services for mentally disordered offenders, resulting in the publication of the *Reed Report*. This made many recommendations to improve the care of all mentally disordered offenders, with special mention of women. It stated that 'in male-dominated environments, women's needs, including their more personal female needs, are liable to be overlooked' (Home Office and Department of Health 1992 p.84). The report emphasizes the importance of services responding to the needs of women and the requirement for different services to those that are tailored to the needs of men. WISH published a report. It states that 'women are currently being cared for in secure settings in which they are marginalized, and which are not designed or equipped to meet their different care, treatment and security needs from men' (Stafford 1999 p.4). This view was reiterated by Dame Rennie Fritchie, the chair of the project group commissioned in 1998 by the High Security Psychiatric Services Commissioning Board (HSPSCB) to investigate improving mental health services for women. This organization noted 'force fitting services for women into a system designed for men does a disservice to women' (HSPSCB 1999 p.iii).

Secure services currently provide adequate care for many male offenders in terms of treatment and protection, for both the patient and the public, particularly by the physical security of the building. However, this does not appear to be the safe and supportive environment that many female patients seem to need. It is probable that staff are able to provide better help for women to deal with many of their problems rather than that provided by the environmental safeguards of fencing or high walls.

More recent reviews into high secure service provision have lead to the Government putting aside £25 million 'to be used in the first instance to facilitate the movement of patients no longer needing high security care' (Department of Health 2000 p.12). This arguably could be describing the women who are placed in inappropriate levels of security. In 1996, figures suggested that '78% of the women in high security settings needed to be in medium security, and 69% in medium secure settings required low security' (Warner and Horn 2001 p.7). The *Tilt Report* (Department of Health 2000 p.13) also recommended that 'the perimeters (of all three special hospitals) should now be enhanced to category B prisons', increasing the physical security of special hospitals and thereby the number of female patients who do not require this level of security.

Many medium secure units are working towards improving the provision of care for women. This includes meeting the requirements set out in the National Service Framework for Mental Health (Department of Health 1999 p.50) of 'achieving fully the patient's charter standard of segregated sleeping, washing and toilet facilities across the NHS'. Some medium secure units favour the setting up of new services, housing the women in completely separate buildings to the men. Others are working towards a dedicated number of beds for female patients in a segregated sleeping area. For some professionals there may be a concern about contagion of undesired behaviours amongst female patients when housed together. Self-harm has been described as a learnt response, but, in my experience, women are able to show support and an enormous degree of empathy for one another during difficult times.

The Multidisciplinary Working Group for Women in Secure Services (MDWGWSS) began meeting at Broadmoor Hospital in 1995 to write some minimum standards of care for women in medium secure settings. This group was put together after it appeared that women, transferred to medium secure units as part of their discharge package from Broadmoor Hospital, were failing to cope in medium security, resulting in a return to high secure services more quickly than their male counterparts. Although this turned out to be untrue, the group's work highlighted the need to look at the standard of care women receive in these settings. They wrote a set of standards (MDWGWSS 1999) which they circulated to all medium secure services along with an audit tool for both staff and patients. It provided a good basis for assessing the provision of quality care for women. At that time the audit showed that many services had much work to do to improve basic standards, such as providing separate bathing facilities. The standards were intended to be used as national guidelines and contain some detail about the minimum provision of therapeutic activities for female patients. The group continues to meet and work on current issues affecting women in medium secure services.

The nature of offences committed by women may seem less severe than those committed by men. Admission to a secure hospital for women is likely to have been precipitated by damage to property, suicidal ideas or incidents of self-harm and acts of aggression or violence towards hospital staff. These incidents are often not pursued to the courts and may not necessarily warrant admission to high secure settings, but they do require high-quality care and treatment. An analysis of the special hospitals case register demonstrated a higher percentage of male patients committed murder, wounding, robbery, rape and indecent assault than their female counterparts (Stafford 1999). In fact many women in secure hospitals are under civil sections of the Mental Health Act (1983) and do not have a forensic history. It seems that as health professionals we find acts of violence and aggression from women more difficult to place in context. Therefore, since service provision for these women has been limited in the past, they have found themselves in high secure hospitals.

A separate but allied issue is the growing numbers of women in prison. A report (Kesteven 2002) commissioned by the National Association for the Care and Resettlement of Offenders highlights that women's offending profile is different to that of men. It notes the particularly high levels of psychiatric morbidity among women prisoners. It recommends that more must be done to reduce the numbers of women being sent to prison and proposes greater use of gender-sensitive, community alternatives rather than custodial sentencing. Additionally, it argues that proper arrangements should be in place for the prompt referral and transfer of prisoners to appropriate secure healthcare settings.

Treatment issues

According to Stafford (1999 p.1), 'women are likely to have a significantly greater history of alcohol misuse or dependency'. Personal experience suggests they are likely to benefit from female-only treatment in this area because men in these settings may be dealing with more drug-related problems, and certainly they describe different reasons driving the cravings. Men tend to talk about self-medication and confidence, for example, whereas women may feel driven to drink in order to cope with the distress of living with abuse.

'Women are also more likely to have been classified as having a personality disorder and meet the diagnostic criteria for borderline personality disorder' (Stafford 1999 p.1). Female patients residing at the Trevor Gibbens Unit have been described as angry, manipulative, threatening, demanding, in need of instant solutions and gratification, and a cause of serious damage to themselves and property. These are words and phrases often associated with bereavement. These emotions and behaviours frequently manifest themselves in explosive situations that need containing by support, staff time and strict adherence to set boundaries and not by high levels of physical security. For example, behavioural care plans, properly drawn up and managed by a psychologist, may be used.

The research states that 'women are significantly more likely to have suffered sexual or physical abuse in childhood, or indeed both' (Stafford 1999 p.1). When placed in a medium secure unit for treatment, women are more often than not in a minority. They are placed within an environment dominated by men, many of whom will also have been abused, and some will have been abusers. People who have been abused may find it difficult to build trusting relationships, and there is always potential for abuse to be re-enacted through sexual harassment or recommitted by actual, physical abuse. Women need to be protected from this, and staff must be aware of the potential damage that can occur when housing women in a mixed environment. Jennings (1994) attempts to compare common practices in psychiatry with early childhood trauma. For example, she compares receiving depot medication with the humiliation of being stripped by an abuser. Or being locked within an institution is compared with being unable to escape a perpetrator's abuse. Occupational therapists often refer to positive role modelling and the therapeutic use of self as an important part of treatment. This necessitates open and consistent strategies for self-reflection, for example, through supervision. A high degree of self-awareness is essential to avoid potentially damaging practice, albeit unwitting or unconscious.

Occupational therapists working closely with women who have survived abuse also need to consider carefully the types of activities on offer. They need to ensure that all staff and patients involved, both male and female, do not take on a negative role model or re-enact the abuse. With careful thought and planning, activities with close physical contact, sporting activities, especially swimming and competitive games can be very positive. Some units have a 'no touch' policy where staff are not permitted to touch patients. However, drawing from personal experience, hugging a patient, under the right circumstances with good boundaries in place, can offer reassurance and allow the patient to encounter positive physical contact. However, occupational therapists do need to feel comfortable offering this and be sure that each individual would view the experience as positive.

'Women are also more likely to be parents than their male counterparts and are perhaps more likely to have been the main carer prior to admission' (Stafford 1999 p.1). Again, staff must have a good understanding of the issues of bereavement surrounding the taking of children into care. Many women feel guilty, inadequate and distraught and are often dealing with the fact that they may never live with their children again. As part of the treatment programme women need to be equipped with parenting skills whatever the future contact with their children. This may involve looking at their own childhood and the parenting they received, since many will have had extremely disrupted childhoods themselves. When considering mothering, there is also the complicated issue of women living alongside other women who may have attempted, or have actually killed, their own or others' children.

Another important consideration for the occupational therapist is that many of the women will have never had a job and, therefore, have been solely dependent on the state for their income. This may lead the occupational therapist to look at issues such as roles, balance of occupations and social issues. They may lack experience of employment because they are younger than their male counterparts. Work experience may be an identified need while in hospital and in the community. They may not be used to mixing and interacting with strangers. Women in society in general are experiencing greater empowerment in life, including better work opportunities, and many are succeeding in bringing up families alongside careers. If we compare this with women in secure services, we need to consider carefully the skills with which we equip female patients. When they leave a forensic environment, they will be re-entering a society where women have more choice in employment. Being a mother, having a job and running a house is hard enough for anyone. Couple that with the stigma of having spent time in a secure hospital and many of the difficulties listed, and the occupational therapist faces a great challenge in preparing women for discharge.

The research carried out on behalf of the HSPSCB asked women what they felt they needed during their period of treatment. The women highlighted 'an increase in responsibility and opportunity to make choices, more information made available to make choices, more female-only activities and more user input and involvement' (HSPSCB 1999 p. 10). User involvement, choice and responsibility are three of the common ways occupational therapists engage patients in treatment. Chacksfield (1997 p. 372) identifies some of the core skills of the occupational therapist working in mental health. These include 'assessment of effect of mental state on activities of daily living, work and leisure; use of activity based group work to enhance cognitive, affective, social, behavioural and life coping skills; observation and monitoring of behaviour to establish risk to self and others and to contribute to the formulation of diagnosis and areas of need'. These skills enable occupational therapists to deliver what women want and this in turn provides a unique opportunity to meet women's needs within a secure environment. The women felt that very few of the activities on offer were 'female orientated, relevant or purposeful and that female activities were restricted because of the needs of the male majority' (HSPSCB, 1999 p.10). For example, many units provide traditionally male-orientated sporting activities or heavy work such as bricklaying, grounds maintenance and woodwork.

Contact with men may be a very significant part of the treatment regime offered to women, but it needs to be carried out under safe circumstances. If possible, it should be a positive experience. On the occasions when it is not, female patients are given an opportunity to process the interactions and put them into the context of their own life experience. Additionally, this provides an opportunity for staff to assess a situation that may mirror future occasions where other female patients may also be at risk. Ascertaining the coping strategies that women employ when faced with uncomfortable or threatening situations provides the therapist with an opportunity to work collaboratively with them to enable new, more appropriate, strategies. This is particularly relevant for the female patient who has been moved from the segregated care of a high secure environment to the mixed environment of medium security. Here some of the therapy is provided within combined sex groups. Reintegration takes place slowly, starting with mixed skills-based groups such as art or cooking, leading to short periods of integrated social time. With support, both men and women build up their confidence and ability to do more therapy-based groups in a mixed setting, but the patient should always be central to deciding the speed of this process. Although the National Service Framework for Mental Health (Department of Health 1999) suggests that some single-sex day space be provided, often women are living within a male-dominated area outside of therapeutic time.

Occupational therapy

So, what exactly should occupational therapists be offering women in secure settings? Treatment should include both individual and group activities that aim to raise self-esteem and give women a positive experience of dealing with relationships. They should build patients' confidence in their abilities to provide stability for any children, whether this is as a provider of care or during visits in in-patient or community placements.

Women who have been abused often have destructive thinking about their bodies, a lack of respect for themselves and may not know how to interact with men without putting themselves at risk. Abuse is often seen in the context of sexual advance and rejection, and all interactions may revolve around these two powerful experiences, making women particularly vulnerable. Experiences living within a mixed-sex environment need to be closely monitored, as abuse can easily be re-enacted during relationships formed with other patients. Women who are scarred from episodes of self-harm may also have issues with their image, and living with men may feed into their feelings of poor self-esteem and lack of confidence. Activities that focus on positive self-image and a healthy interest in appearance provide not only an opportunity to deal with these issues but also informal opportunities for women to bond and support one another. Activities as simple as nail painting, for example, bring together women who may feel they have very little in common. The women leave the room feeling they have been viewed as important human beings that are worth pampering. They have also spent time thinking about their appearance in a simple, non-threatening way. Allowing the women to paint the nails of staff has boosted their confidence and self-esteem and breaks down the staff–patient relationship in a safe way. Touch of hand and nails can be a safe part of the body for many women and does not carry the same degree of risk of causing distress as some other activities like, for instance, massage.

Women also have very different health needs to men and are entitled to education, access to advice and treatment for female-related physical health problems. They should also be receiving information on any annual or regular health screens which should not be discussed in a mixed health-education group, allowing the women to ask personal questions pertinent to their own situation if required.

Other activities and groups include leisure groups, relaxation, skill-based groups such as anger management, anxiety management, problem-solving and coping strategies. Groups that allow women to express themselves, perhaps using talking therapy or creative techniques, or a combination of both, are also important. Discussion groups to look at women's issues and roles are popular. Some services have set up self-harm groups to focus specifically on this behaviour in women.

A combination of health and beauty issues within a group setting has worked well with women in the Trevor Gibbens Unit, who, as one patient put it, 'enjoyed the opportunity to do "girlie" things whilst learning about taking care of themselves'. From the therapist's point of view there was a noticeable difference in confidence and appearance within the ward environment generally. These women also seemed to enjoy very practical sessions such as cookery, where the majority felt able to excel in an activity that would certainly be of relevance to most when discharged. Shopping trips are also extremely popular and have been requested again and again. One lady was heard to comment that 'it was so nice to go out as a group of women,' and, 'I haven't had that much fun in years'. It also provided the therapist with an opportunity to look at health issues, budgeting and social skills during what can be construed as a very normal activity for women.

Sport has long been identified as an activity that is highly beneficial to people with both physical and mental health problems, and certainly within a forensic environment is well recognized as a therapeutic tool for all patients. While some female patients will happily join in five-a-side football with the male patients, others will prefer women-only sport, and certainly a female escort is necessary for any integrated team games. However, a healthy sense of rivalry and competition between men and women may seem natural, and therefore integrated activities can be encouraged when appropriate. Leisure activities within the community require a careful balance of male and female staff, for example a male escort should never be left in the position of escorting a woman in the swimming pool. Initial trips to such places are carefully monitored, as reintegration with the public in general can be stressful when compared with the careful, slow reintegration with male patients in the relative safety of a forensic unit. Women with a history of eating disorders such as anorexia nervosa need a carefully monitored exercise programme that encourages gentle cardiovascular exercise for general health and well-being. Some women experience weight gain because of side effects of psychotropic medication, and this should be handled in a sensitive manner with a well-monitored exercise programme. Many forensic services are lucky enough to have a small gym on site and will be able to offer this kind of intervention at many stages of treatment. At times, it has been necessary to consider issues around appropriate clothing when trying to involve female patients in using sports facilities. Women may need encouragement to wear appropriate, supportive clothing, particularly if the activity is integrated with male staff or patients.

Experience of work may benefit not only those women who have never been employed but also those who have. In the Trevor Gibbens Unit there is a strong culture of patients being involved in work which benefits those living there (for example daily cleaning of the patients' kitchen, emptying the ashtrays, cleaning the unit cars, etc.). All patients are given the opportunity to hold a job and alongside the financial gain comes responsibility, accountability, a sense of achievement, increased confidence and ability to perform to a standard acceptable to others. The female patients are encouraged to take jobs of all types and not just those that were perhaps viewed as traditional to the female role. This fits with the current culture of women beginning to work in male-orientated jobs and perhaps gives the female patients some experience of the difficulties this can pose. The unit is in the process of extending these work opportunities, for women, into the wider community. Until this is well established, all discharged patients have the opportunity initially to continue with some form of work at the Unit if this is assessed as being beneficial.

Conclusion

It seems that the type of offences, personal background and diagnoses are the key factors which make women housed in secure services different to men. These factors should be taken into consideration when planning services and intervention. An occupational therapist aims to empower a patient to live life to their maximum capability. Through provision of practical skills and treatment, which acknowledges loss and trauma, women can be enabled to continue life successfully outside of secure settings. For the occupational therapist this is achieved by responding to female patients who themselves identify 'the need to engage in purposeful and relevant activities' (HSPSCB 1999 p.10).

References

Chacksfield J (1997) Forensic occupational therapy: is it a developing specialism? British Journal of Therapy and Rehabilitation 4(7) 371–374.

Department of Health and Home Office (1992) Review of Health and Social Services for Mentally Disordered Offenders and Others Requiring Similar Services, chaired by Dr John Reed. Final Summary Report. London: HMSO.

Department of Health (1999) National Service Framework for Mental Health. London: Department of Health.

Department of Health (2000) Report of the Review of Security at the High Secure Hospitals, chaired by Sir Richard Tilt. London: HMSO.

High Secure Psychiatric Services Commissioning Board (1999) Secure Futures for Women. London: Department of Health.

Jennings A (1994) On being invisible in the mental health system. Journal of Mental Health Administration 21(4) 374–387.

Kesteven S (2002) Women who Challenge: Women Offenders and Mental Health Issues. A Nacro Policy Report. London: National Association for the Care and Resettlement of Offenders.

MDWGWSS (1999) Minimum Standards of Care for Women in Secure Settings, chaired by S Pearson. Unpublished: Broadmoor Hospital, Crowthorne.

Mental Health Act (1983) London: HMSO.

Stafford P (1999) Defining Gender Issue: Redefining Women's Services. London: Women in Special Hospitals.

Warner S and Horn R (2001) Introduction: Positive directions for women in secure environments. Issues in Forensic Psychology (2) 6–10.

CHAPTER 16

Forensic occupational therapy within learning disability services

RACHEL PRENTICE AND KIRSTY WILSON

Introduction

Ward (1990 p.4) describes the learning-disabled individual as one whose 'intellectual functioning is significantly below average and having marked impairment in the ability to adapt to the cultural demands of society'. When offending behaviour is also apparent, such an individual may find themselves in a forensic psychiatric setting. This chapter is based on experience gained at Langdon Hospital's Leander Unit in Devon. Leander is a 37-bed regional open forensic psychiatric unit for people with mild and borderline learning disabilities. It consists of a 16-bed admission ward with an extra care area and a 16-bed rehabilitation/pre-discharge ward. In addition, there is a training flat staffed between the hours of 9 and 5 for supported independent living and five additional self-contained flats. The Leander Unit provides a service to both male and female patients, and nursing staff are trained in both mental health and mental handicap care.

Detention

As in any other forensic setting patients are detained under part II and part III of the Mental Health Act (1983). Commonly, this is under Section 3 and Sections 37/41 respectively. In addition, the forensic learning-disabled patient may be detained on bail assessment or probation order. Typically, the patient will be on remand and a referral will be made to the forensic learning disability service from a solicitor, court, prison or locality team. An assessment will be conducted jointly by the consultant and another member of the team, often a nurse. If it is felt that a placement in the hospital is appropriate, a recommendation will be forwarded to the court. If the court is agreeable, the patient will be admitted for a further period of assessment while on bail. This will usually take place during a three-month period, and the multidisciplinary team will then collaborate in order to make further recommendations to the court. Following the assessment period, if it is believed that the patient would benefit from a longer period of hospitalization, the court may recommend a period of probation for two to three years. This will include an initial condition of hospital residency. In practice, the patient is likely to serve 18 months to two years of the probation order in hospital. For patients resident on Leander's admission and rehabilitation wards, the average length of stay is 17.2 months. Following discharge, the remainder of the order is spent in the community under the supervision of the probation service. This marks out the learning-disabled forensic service as being quite distinct from general forensic settings.

A brief overview of the literature points to general agreement that the learning-disabled population should be in receipt of a specialist service, distinct from that provided for those with clear mental illness as their primary diagnosis. Also, severe learning disability and mild/moderate learning disability require different management strategies (Cohen and Eastman 2000, Gralton et al. 2000, Halstead 1996 and Johnson et al. 1993).

General presentation

Many patients have multiple diagnoses. Mental illness, genetic disorders and pervasive developmental disorders are common diagnoses made in addition to that of learning disability. Gralton et al. (2000) highlight that population surveys suggest an increased prevalence of schizophrenia in the learning-disabled population. They detail six case reports where treatment for schizophrenia markedly improved the clinical picture for learning-disabled patients. Fraser and Nolan (1994) (cited by Dickens 1998) suggest that prevalence of mental illness within the population of learning-disabled people ranges from 8% to 15% with regard to serious disorders, but with the inclusion of minor disorders the incidence may rise to over 50%. Similarly, Dickens (1998) notes that autism is a common concurrent condition. Many patients, while not having full-blown autism, present with autistic spectrum disorders. Asperger's syndrome is a diagnosis not uncommon on the Leander Unit.

Without wishing to generalize the needs of the forensic learning-disabled population, there are common areas of need and these are summarized in Table 16.1 (below). This demonstrates that there are clear parallels between a client group with a primary diagnosis of mental illness and those with a primary diagnosis of borderline learning disability; however, there are also some notable differences.

A strength of patients with a diagnosis of borderline learning disability is high motivation. This may be due in part to an absence of negative symptoms associated with mental illness. Uptake of groups and therapy sessions is high, with consistent attendance. Personal experience suggests

Table 16.1 Common areas of need

Behavioural/Social Performance	Cognitive
Restlessness/hyperactivity	Deficits re comprehension, logic and reasoning
Immature behaviour and verbal interactions	Poor educational achievements
Poor interpersonal functioning	Lack of insight and self-awareness
Inability to recognize and respond to social cues	Limited attention span
Lack of adaptive coping strategies	Egocentricity
Reliance on maladaptive strategies	Low self-esteem
	Cognitive rigidity

this may sometimes be the desire to gain a certificate of attendance, or coffee and a jaffa cake, rather than a desire to change behaviour. However, whatever the initial motivating factor, patients soon welcome the opportunity to develop their skills and abilities and voice pride in their achievements. One patient, who has actively participated in user activities since admission, takes his role of patient representative very seriously. He thrives on the responsibility and takes great pride in keeping his file of minutes in good order, despite being unable to read. A combination of a nurturing approach along with an expressed belief in their potential enable patients to mature and develop.

The occupational therapy role

As with any other area of healthcare, the successful team will work together, sharing information and supporting one another to carry out their unique function within the team, to achieve an holistic package of care for each individual. Essentially, the role of the occupational therapist with the forensic learning-disabled population is the same as that within forensic psychiatry in general. It is, however, the acknowledgement of the clients' special limitations and how these influence and inform practice that adds a different dimension.

Typically, the occupational therapist will perform a role that includes educator, clinician, advocate and facilitator. The White Paper *Valuing People: A New Strategy for Learning Disability* (Department of Health 2001) highlights the four key principles of *rights*, *independence*, *choice* and *inclusion*. These principles lie at the heart of the Government's proposals aimed at providing opportunities for those with learning disabilities, and their families, to live full and independent lives. These same principles are, and have long been, at the heart of the occupational therapy profession and naturally influence practice within forensic learning disability settings.

Theoretical approaches to practice

Drawing from experience, it is strongly recommended that occupational therapy models are observed. In the Leander Unit, aspects of both Reed and Sanderson's (1992) 'Adaptation through Occupation Model' and Kielhofner's (1995) 'Model of Human Occupation' (MoHO) are regularly applied. An eclectic approach to practice should not be viewed as a lack of understanding of theory leading to a haphazard approach to care. Rather, in the authors' experience, it is helpful to extract and apply elements from different models according to the specific needs presented by the patient.

Often within learning disability services a behavioural approach forms the basis of interventions, with the aim of promoting desired behaviours while seeking to reduce or eliminate problematic or undesirable behaviours. Occupational therapists will be familiar with the process of writing behavioural objectives with clear measurable outcomes.

Cognitive behavioural approaches are becoming more commonplace and used widely within group work with this client group. Difficulties though may be experienced with a cognitive approach if there are expectations that the individual can articulate their thoughts and feelings readily.

Using a client-centred approach the patient is asked to prioritize areas of need and agree targets, or goals, based on these priorities or perceived areas of need. The assumption here is that motivation to engage in the therapeutic process is therefore assured. It may be that, within a learning disability setting, suggested goals highlight a lack of self-awareness, and there may be conflict between the client's goals and the therapist's goals. Sensitivity in approach is key where such discrepancies occur.

Assessment

Assessment of an individual with a mild or borderline learning disability who has offended and may also have a mental illness is complex. The occupational therapist needs to establish a full and accurate understanding of the patient's occupational performance through a detailed analysis of their functional abilities and deficits.

For the **initial assessment**, relevant background information is gathered prior to meeting with the patient. This includes:

- reason for admission, index offence and diagnosis
- forensic history
- psychiatric history

- medical history
- personal and family history
- drug and alcohol history
- risk assessment.

The next step in assessment is **establishing rapport**. Flexibility and sensitivity are needed when building a therapeutic relationship with this client group, who have found themselves in a new and unfamiliar environment and may not have full insight and understanding into their reason for admission. Many patients come from abusive (physical, sexual and emotional) or dysfunctional backgrounds and may have difficulty opening up to and trusting new people.

A **full functional assessment** can occur only when a reasonable level of trust has been established. A full and comprehensive assessment may take several weeks to complete. The aim is to identify occupational performance and areas of occupational dysfunction, particularly where this has contributed to offending or problematic behaviour. It includes exploration of:

- occupational roles, interests and values
- occupational balance
- the patient's level of satisfaction with their lifestyle prior to admission
- the patient's current performance skills.

This provides a baseline from which further assessment and intervention can be planned.

Various **assessment tools** and methods may be used. On the Leander Unit, interviews, checklists, questionnaires, observations and standardized assessments are all utilized. This is because a flexible approach when administering assessments is needed with this client group. Formerly, occupational therapy departments frequently devised their own assessments because of a lack of assessment tools developed for use in learning disabilities. Using an occupational therapy model helps to ensure a full and holistic assessment is undertaken. This theoretical framework influences the choice of assessment tools. Role and interest checklist, the Canadian Occupational Performance Measure (COPM) (Law et al. 1994), the Assessment of Motor and Process Skills (AMPS) (Fisher 1999) and other MoHO assessments have all been successfully used at the Leander Unit.

Intervention

Occupational therapists **select activities** to which the patient attaches some meaning or value (purposeful activity) and use core professional skills of analysing, grading, adapting and applying purposeful activities to bring about change and remedy dysfunction. Hagedorn (1995) describes this in detail. One of the skills of the occupational therapist working in forensic learning disability is to identify and understand how a patient's needs and limitations have contributed to their offending behaviour. By planning and implementing intervention to address dysfunction, the therapist is trying to develop the patient's occupational skills and functional independence. This is no different to all other areas of occupational therapy, but, in forensic learning disabilities, occupational therapy is also contributing to the process of addressing and preventing offending behaviour.

Planning intervention is a skilled task. The formulation of a rehabilitation plan is achieved through interpretation and analysis of data gathered during assessment. The many and complex needs and deficits presented by the forensic learning-disabled patient are prioritized and incorporated into realistic and appropriate short-, medium- and long-term goals. It is essential to work collaboratively with the patient when agreeing and setting goals so that their needs and wishes can be taken into account. However, the therapist may need to take more of a directive role depending on the patient's attitude and insight into their needs.

Occupational therapy in this field should incorporate the following **interventions** and the case study on page 169 puts them in context.

- activities of daily living, personal and domestic
- the development of leisure interests and hobbies
- vocational rehabilitation
- the development of social skills and appropriate behaviour
- building self-worth and self-esteem
- the development of community skills, e.g. budgeting, shopping, road safety, accessing community resources
- the development of cognitive skills
- the development of coping skills, particularly flexible thinking, problem-solving, anxiety and anger management.

Some may challenge the place of direct interventions to address cognitive-skills deficits within the occupational therapy role, as they are not traditional activity-based interventions. However, occupational therapists are well placed to facilitate these interventions within the total rehabilitation programme. The emphasis is to develop positive coping skills, increasing the patient's functional independence, thus decreasing their reliance on negative coping strategies, like antisocial and criminal behaviours, and prevent reoffending or social isolation. Occupational therapists not only enable patients to develop a knowledge base regarding positive coping skills and strategies; they can also enable patients to apply and develop these skills during practical and realistic situations in the hospital and in the community. It is acknowledged that other professions, particularly psychology, have expertise in this area, and working together to provide interventions is certainly recommended. This can be very successful and has the knock-on effect of enhancing team working, which can only benefit patient care.

Physical health issues may need to be addressed, for example with the older long-stay patient, and smoking-related illnesses are common. The presentation of motor and perceptual problems are sometimes apparent, particularly 'clumsiness', coordination difficulties and spatial awareness problems.

A decision regarding the appropriateness of group-based or individual intervention will be based on the patient's needs identified during the assessment. Individual intervention and group work are both used with this client group. It cannot be assumed that the provision of intervention to the forensic learning-disabled population will be uniform or identical. Patients frequently benefit from involvement in both types of therapy. This may be by using a combination of group and individual intervention at the same time or by using one as a lead into the other. Owing to cognitive limitations, greater learning may result from individually tailored packages as some information loss can occur in group settings. However, experience suggests that experiential learning has the more powerful retentive potential and can occur more readily in group settings. Others have noted that 'people with learning disabilities may have pockets of particular skills that are not reflective of their overall performance. For this reason the mix of experiential and skills-based learning is particularly effective within the field of learning disabilities' (Creek 2002 p.427).

Special considerations when working in forensic learning disability services

Firm boundaries

Firm boundaries must be established and maintained by all staff. Patients frequently present with problem behaviours, such as verbal and physical aggression and low tolerance to frustration (Johnson et al. 1993). By setting and reinforcing limits on what is and is not acceptable behaviour, problem behaviours can be managed and over time, it is hoped, decrease.

Consistency

A consistent approach from all staff is essential. Regular and effective communication between professionals will ensure a consistent and collaborative approach and prevent professionals from carrying out conflicting interventions.

Limitations

It is important to take into account the patient's cognitive abilities, in particular intellectual and language abilities. Limitations in cognitive functioning greatly affect the patient's ability to understand, to learn and to communicate effectively. Patients frequently learn to compensate for their limitations and will appear to understand when the reality is they are confused and may be misinterpreting language. This brings about several implications for practice. First, it is important to be aware and sensitive to the language used when orally communicating with patients. Clear and simple language is best. It is often helpful to ask the patient to repeat back information to ensure they have thoroughly understood and taken on board what has been said. Second, the helpfulness and appropriateness of using written materials during intervention must be evaluated, particularly the use of handouts, flip charts and overheads in group work. If a patient has no, or a very low, measurable reading and writing age, these will be of little use. Visual aids and cues are generally found to be of more use than written materials. Creativity, therefore, is clearly needed in order to provide an effective service.

Evaluation

Evaluation is a continuous process occurring throughout the occupational therapy process. Rehabilitation plans are reviewed and modified in conjunction with the patient. The patient will change and progress throughout their rehabilitation; however, the rate of change varies with each individual. Subtle, yet significant, changes will be occurring, and regular evaluation is essential in order to identify these changes. Multidisciplinary review and evaluation, usually through the care programme approach, occurs every three months. This not only allows an evaluation of each discipline's intervention but also is a forum for planning the next stage of rehabilitation, thus maintaining a future focus.

Discharge planning

Discharge planning is carried out in conjunction with locality teams and those responsible for ongoing care. Regular liaison enables a comprehensive handover of recommendations regarding ongoing areas of need and interventions, along with a summary of treatment and progress to date. The occupational therapist may assist with the transition between hospital and community by visiting accommodation and occupational facilities with the patient. This makes it sound easy but, in practice, transfer can be difficult. Halstead (1996 p. 81) highlights that forensic learning-disabled patients fit 'so many borderlines that no service is willing to take them on'.

Difficulties can occur in finding a locality team to take responsibility for these patients, owing to their multiple diagnoses. Conflict may exist as to whether a mental health or learning disability service is best placed to manage patients' ongoing care.

Case Study

Ted, aged 26, was admitted from prison on a bail assessment with charges of criminal damage. A three-year probation order, with condition of hospital residency, followed a two-month assessment period at Langdon Hospital. He was known to local learning disability services. Four years earlier he was subject to a two-year probation order for assault and a public-order offence. Background history revealed Ted was taken into care when he was 4 years old. He had foster placements until the age of 18 but later maintained no significant contact with his biological or foster families. He attended a special school until aged 16. He left with no qualifications. From the age of 18, he lived in a variety of residential care homes, bed and breakfasts and an independent flat. These placements broke down due to loss of temper, property damage and assaultive behaviour. Ted had no previous paid employment, though for two years he did part-time voluntary work.

His occupational therapy initial assessment revealed Ted had an accurate grasp of the reasons for his admission to hospital. Ted's stated aims for intervention were:

* to be independent
* to learn to control his temper
* to do voluntary work.

Aims identified by the occupational therapist included:

* improve his coping skills, such as anger management and anxiety management
* develop his cognitive abilities, for example improving memory concentration and minimizing cognitive rigidity
* increase Ted's self-confidence/esteem
* develop his independent living skills
* increase his range of leisure interests
* improve his social support networks
* provide opportunities for Ted to develop his employment skills
* promote his skills in self-expression and communication.

Ted was resident on the admission ward for six months, during which time he engaged in groups and individual sessions, as outlined in Table 16.2.

Table 16.2 Admission ward intervention

Intervention	Aims
Hobbies group	to promote leisure interests to encourage social interaction to build self-esteem/confidence
Social skills group	to learn and rehearse skills and build confidence in ability to initiate and maintain social relationships
Individual cookery	to develop domestic skills to develop cognitive skills, e.g. memory, concentration, problem-solving to encourage self-esteem
Anger management group and 1-to-1 psychology	to promote recognition of anger triggers and existing coping mechanisms to replace maladaptive coping strategies with adaptive ones ongoing monitoring of application of techniques learnt
Anxiety management	to understand causes and personal symptoms of anxiety to develop effective management techniques

His progress was monitored, and a general improvement in mood and self-esteem was noted. Ted was felt to have made headway in the social skills group, and it was agreed to refer him to a subsequent, more complex, block of social skills training following transfer to the rehabilitation ward. He was observed to manage several threatening situations with other patients well, and no aggressive or inappropriate behaviours were reported. Steady improvements in expressing his needs appropriately were seen. Following transfer to the rehabilitation ward, where Ted was resident for 11 months, he attended groups and sessions as outlined in Table 16.3.

In addition to this, Ted had access to education, speech therapy, physical health and fitness (physiotherapy) and maintained contact with psychology, individual cookery sessions and hobbies group. He continued to actively engage in his rehabilitation programme and remained motivated, pleasant on approach and to have a clear future orientation. Individual life skills intervention, social skills and self-esteem groups made some impact on his reported levels of anxiety regarding his return to the community, although he continued to approach new situations with concrete expectations. With regard to vocational rehabilitation, he demonstrated the ability to cope with most basic tasks set and to seek help or advice appropriately and when necessary, indicating a level of

Table 16.3 Rehabilitation ward intervention

Intervention	Aims
Problem-solving groups	to promote flexible thinking and reduce cognitive rigidity to learn positive coping strategies to deal with problems to allow practical application of learned skills
Self-esteem group	to build on improvements in self-esteem seen through engagement in group work since admission
Individual life skills	to build familiarity and confidence in accessing community resources
Personal relationships	to promote awareness, understanding and discussion of issues pertaining to the development of physical/sexual relationships, to include safe sex, legal issues and emotional implications
Vocational rehabilitation	to carry out a full assessment of work skills, attitudes and behaviours to provide opportunity to re-engage in work habits and routines and maintain interest in future work opportunities
Social skills group	to learn and rehearse skills and build confidence in ability to initiate and maintain social relationships

insight into his own limitations. Four months prior to discharge, Ted was referred to the training flat to further develop his independent living skills. He attended on a daily basis and was supported to take responsibility for shopping and cooking his own meals within a limited budget.

As plans for discharge were formulated, his ongoing needs were identified as:

* cognitive rigidity demonstrated in difficulties with problem-solving and flexible thinking
* further development of coping strategies including anger and anxiety management and assertion training.

Seventeen months after admission, Ted was discharged, and responsibility was handed to the community learning disability team and the probation service for the remainder of his probation order. He was placed in supported accommodation, where he was expected to live semi-independently and take responsibility for most aspects of activities of daily living. He was referred to a local sheltered work facility with opportunities for community work placements.

Conclusion

In summary, we hope that this chapter has highlighted the importance of a robust assessment process as the basis for tailoring personalized rehabilitative activities for a unique client group with complex needs. Occupational therapy is clearly central to the rehabilitation process within forensic learning disability. The needs and challenges presented by this client group provide us, as therapists, with ongoing opportunities to utilize our extensive skills, knowledge and creativity to the full. We also hope we have been able to share some of our enthusiasm and professional satisfaction, gained by working in this particular specialism within the field of forensic psychiatry.

References and further reading

Attwood T (1998) Asperger's Syndrome: A Guide for Parents and Professionals. London: Jessica Kingsley Publishers.

Cohen A and Eastman N (2000) Assessing Forensic Mental Health Need, Policy, Theory and Research. London: Gaskell.

Creek J (ed.) (2002) Occupational Therapy and Mental Health (3rd edition). Edinburgh: Churchill Livingstone.

Department of Health (2001) Valuing People: A New Strategy for Learning Disability for the Twenty-first Century (White Paper). London: HMSO.

Dickens D (1998) 'Learning Disability'. In: The Special Hospitals in Managing High Security Psychiatric Care, Kaye C and Franey A (eds.). London: Jessica Kingsley Publishers.

Fisher A (1999) Assessment of Motor and Process Skills (3rd edition). Colorado: Three Star Press.

Gralton E, James A and Crocombe J (2000) The diagnosis of schizophrenia in the borderline learning-disabled population. Six case reports. Journal of Forensic Psychiatry 11(1) 185–187.

Hagedorn R (1995) Occupational Therapy: Perspectives and Processes. Edinburgh: Churchill Livingstone.

Hagedorn R (1997) Foundations for Practice in Occupational Therapy (2nd edition). Edinburgh: Churchill Livingstone.

Halstead S (1996) Forensic psychiatry for people with learning disability. Advances in Psychiatric Treatment 2(2) 76–85.

Johnson C, Smith J, Stainer G and Donovan M (1993) Mildly mentally handicapped offenders: An alternative to custody. Psychiatric Bulletin 17(4) 199–201.

Kielhofner G (ed.) (1995) Model of Human Occupation: Theory and Application (2nd edition). Baltimore: Williams and Wilkins.

Law M, Baptiste S, Carswell A, McColl M, Polatajko H, Pollock N (1994) Canadian Occupational Performance Measure. Toronto: Canadian Association of Occupational Therapists.

Reed K and Sanderson S (1992) Concepts of Occupational Therapy. Baltimore: Williams and Wilkins.

Ward A (1990) The Power to Act. Glasgow: Scottish Society for the Mentally Handicapped.

CHAPTER 17
Self-injury or relief from overwhelming emotions

ANN McQUE

Introduction

Cutting up. Deliberate self-harm. Parasuicide. Are you familiar with these dramatic words that are often used and elicit strong emotions? How do they make you feel when you hear them? It may be shock, abhorrence, anger or disbelief; it certainly is for many people. Occupational therapists believe themselves to be holistic carers who can be advocates for their patients and clients; however, if they are to care for those who suffer with this presentation, they must first explore their own reactions and feelings. It is vital for carers to understand that their negative reactions can only reinforce the belief of the individual that they are worthless or disgusting.

Our ideas of what is self-injury are culturally based. To Western eyes the binding of children's feet in China, or the alteration of head shape by the ancient Egyptians for aesthetic reasons, may appear barbaric. However, these are among the more well-known of many body-changing customs and rituals carried out throughout history. To some people, the modern fashion for body piercing could be added to this list. The difference between these customs and self-harm is that they were, or are, socially acceptable. Mutilation is also a central theme in many religions including Christianity. Matthew 5:29-30 directs Christians to 'pluck out an offending eye', or 'cut off an offending hand, rather than being cast whole into hell'. There are recorded instances of self-mutilation in the animal kingdom, especially among primates held in captivity.

Definition

There appears to be no universally accepted terminology for self-harming behaviours. However, for the purposes of this discussion, we shall divide it into three categories:

- self-mutilation
- suicide
- self-injury.

173

'In **self-mutilation** the stated intention is often to rid oneself of an offending organ or body part, typically one to which one's culture attributes moral qualities (such as evil eye, filthy tongue, genitalia)' (Tantam and Whittaker 1992 p. 452). Self-mutilation is rare and is usually performed only by those who are psychotic, intoxicated with drugs or suffer organic brain syndrome (Favazza 1989). In these cases, there is an element of punishment or atonement for sins, heavenly commands or demonic influence.

Suicide is different from other self-harming behaviours in that at least part of the person wants to die at the time of harming. It should also be remembered that there could also be deaths from self-injury that have gone wrong rather than an intention to die. Suicide is not usually caused by one factor alone but by an accumulation of difficulties over time. Risk factors may include:

- psychiatric illnesses, especially depression
- substance misuse
- social isolation
- loss or separation.

Some people who self-injure eventually do attempt, or commit, suicide; research suggests that as many as 10% of patients admitted to hospital following self-harm commit suicide within ten years (Levi 1998). All of these factors are present in forensic settings and therefore the risk of suicide is high.

For convenience, all self-harming behaviours of a culturally or socially unacceptable nature and without conscious suicidal intent are grouped under the heading of **self-injury**. The most common injuries include skin cutting 72%, skin burning 35%, self-hitting 30%, interference with wound healing and skin scratching 22% (Favazza and Conterio 1989). These proportions appear to have remained static since this original research. The inclusion of substance misuse and eating disorders as self-injury is controversial, but it does appear that self-harm can at least alternate with these disorders and they often have the same pathology. There are also people who provoke others to inflict the harm by inciting violence against them, for example, by deliberately starting a fight in order to be beaten up. The extreme version of this scenario is what in America is called 'Death by Cop' where the individual stage-manages an incident which leaves the police no alternative but to shoot that person.

Self-injury does not only occur within psychiatric conditions or in forensic settings. Many people with otherwise successful lives self-injure. Where it does occur, in mental health, common consent suggests that the most prevalent diagnosis for those self-harming is borderline personality disorder or other flamboyant personality disorders (histrionic, narcissistic), post-traumatic stress disorder and depression. There is also a close association with dissociative identity disorder (formally known as multiple personality disorder) and childhood sexual or physical abuse (Tantam and Whittaker 1992).

Delinquent adolescents and incarcerated adults are considered to be at greater risk of self-harm because it is thought that confinement may provoke self-harming behaviour (Haines et al. 1995). Therefore, the forensic services will experience a higher incidence than in the general population. It is also likely that individual incidents are at the extreme end of the spectrum of self-injuring behaviours and to be of a more bizarre form. In the past, forensic staff used all means, including restraint and seclusion, to try to prevent individuals from harming themselves. This proved to be virtually impossible, as the ingenuity of the individual who wants to self-harm is boundless. There is even anecdotal evidence of a high secure patient using crisps to disembowel himself (one of the old Broadmoor legends), but it is certainly true that paint chipped from the wall or window frame makes a good cutting tool.

Today the emphasis is on preventing serious harm and for the patient to take responsibility, whenever possible, for the care of their own wounds. Outside the forensic setting there is a strong movement, among those who self-harm, to keep special equipment especially for the purpose of self-harm, as well as first-aid materials to treat the wound and avoid further damage by preventing infection. This has proved to be liberating for many people, helping them to harm themselves less. This becomes more difficult where there is a risk that either the individual or a third party could use it for the harm of others.

Why do people self-injure?

The most common reasons for self-harm cited by researchers, carers and those who self-harm are threefold:

* a coping strategy
* titillation
* communication/attracting attention.

If we look at **coping strategy** it can be seen as 'a purposeful, if morbid, act of self-help' (Favazza 1989), a way to live with overwhelming emotional pain. Many factors can be involved in the circumstances that lead to self-injury as a way of coping. In a secure hospital setting it may then become the act of taking back control, in a prison it becomes an act of defiance or simply a way of venting anger and frustration. It can relieve the symptoms of depersonalization, that is feelings of unreality or separation of mind and body. Patients have described how the flow of blood will release inner tension, stop racing thoughts or reverse feelings of deadness and detachment from reality. As one patient said, 'Cutting makes me feel human again.' In many cases, it is the use of physical pain to provide relief from overwhelming emotions.

Titillation or sensation-seeking tend to be the preserve of those with an impulsive personality, giving them feelings of euphoria. It may include instances of substance misuse and bulimia. This type of self-injury is sometimes thought of and treated as addiction.

Communication/attracting attention can be seen in a number of ways: as a cry for help, a need for support, manipulation or emotional blackmail. Everybody needs attention! Self-injury is often a desperate attempt to draw attention to distress and its causes. Many sufferers cannot, or have never been allowed to, express their needs and feelings (big boys don't cry), therefore they do not know other ways to communicate them. As one client explained, 'Self-injury is my only relief from overwhelming emotions'. It is important to remember that many of the patients seen by forensic occupational therapists have histories of loss. Loss of control, self-esteem, roles, relationships and for two groups (those with borderline personality disorder and sufferers of childhood abuse) probably a loss of their childhood too. Although many people think of self-injury as a female trait, both men and women self-injure. Some research even suggests that it is more common among men but that more women receive psychological help (Tantam and Whittaker 1992). Another report suggests that self-injury is more common in women, reflecting the different pressures and expectations between men and women in our society (Arnold and Babiker 1998). When men self-injure, it is usually where they have less power (such as when in prison).

Reactions to self-injury

In a forensic setting, occupational therapists will normally work as part of a multidisciplinary team. This is doubly important when working with self-injuring behaviour where consistency of approach is vital. All members of the team need to be aware of their own feelings and reactions, because self-injury commonly arouses uncomfortable feelings and reactions in workers. These are described as:

- shock, horror and disgust
- incomprehension
- fear and anxiety
- distress and sadness
- anger and frustration
- powerlessness and inadequacy.

(Arnold and Babika 1998)

This then leads to unhelpful responses such as condemnatory attitudes or authoritarian approaches. There is anecdotal evidence that the treatment received by some individuals, when presenting with self-injury in Accident and Emergency Departments is of hostility, more pain infliction and being made to wait inordinate lengths of time for treatment. All of which only serve to reinforce the feelings of worthlessness leading to greater self-injuring behaviour and may lead to statements such as, 'I had to learn to scream silently'(Pembroke 1994 p.32). One way for the therapist to deal with personal feelings, reactions or emotional issues is to maintain a diary. This can be used in good and supportive clinical supervision, which should always be sought by those working with emotional issues. Although it is statistically more likely that instances of self-injury will happen outside of therapy activities, it is very important that occupational therapists are part of the shared plan for dealing with any incidents that do occur.

A number of studies have identified evenings as the most likely time for self-injury. This may indicate that structured activity has a part to play in reducing incidences of self-injury. Studies by Hemkendreis (1992), Garner et al. (1994) and Walsh (2000), however, did not produce any correlation between patterns of structured activity and patterns of self-injury. This does not mean that occupational therapists do not have important skills to offer in the treatment of patients who self-harm. In fact, the skills of occupational therapists seem to be almost tailor made for this client group, particularly when a client-centred holistic approach is used. The areas identified as the reasons for self-harming include loss of self-esteem, roles, control and a sense of powerlessness. These are all areas in which occupational therapists have specialist skills. For this reason, it is usual for the occupational therapist to concentrate on the here-and-now element of any treatment plan for this client group, unless they have specific skills in another area, such as counselling.

There are several websites relating to self-injury. These may be suitable for some clients in the community to access directly, although any professional should investigate sites before recommending them. As an example, www.selfinjury.freeserve.co.uk is a useful site written collaboratively by people who self-injure and the Bristol Crisis Service for Women.

Integral to the work of the forensic mental health team is risk assessment. The forensic occupational therapist will always need to undertake a thorough risk assessment on both the possible activities and the patient before any treatment plan is agreed. The occupational therapy department will contain many objects that could be used for either self-harm or suicide. It is for this reason, as well as for the protection of others, that a good system of tool and other dangerous substances checks must be instituted.

Occupational therapy programme

Not all patients will require the same occupational therapy interventions, and any treatment plan will be individual to, and agreed with, that person. It may be useful to look at some individual experiences in order to see how such a treatment plan might be used. An initial occupational therapy programme is likely to include self-esteem activities as a high priority because, as already stated, poor self-esteem and feelings of worthlessness are common in this client group. It is therefore important to break the cycle of 'I am worthless, therefore I self-injure, which proves that I am worthless'. Jane provides one example of how a first intervention was achieved.

Case example

Jane, a young woman aged 20, was admitted to a high secure hospital following an index offence of attempted murder. Her father had sexually abused her as a child, and she now has a history of self-injury using cigarettes to burn in a grid, of six across by eight down, on her forearm. Her expressed reasons for this self-injury were of guilt and worthlessness. Jane was resistant to taking part in any activities but was eventually persuaded to attend the pottery group where slip casting was used with a mould to produce ornaments. The second process of painting the ornament was used as the initial activity for Jane, providing her with a successful outcome. As it was close to Christmas, Jane had chosen to make a child playing with snowballs as her project. On returning to the ward with it, she asked a nurse for materials to wrap it up to send to a friend as a Christmas present. The nurse asked who had made it. 'I did,' replied Jane straightening up as she said it. 'Really?' said the nurse as she called others to see. Everyone admired the ornament and then someone asked Jane to make one for her. By this time, Jane appeared to have grown six inches. This was not contrived action by the staff but a genuine reaction to an activity that was originally only expected to increase self-esteem through Jane discovering that she could be successful.

The next, or intermediate plan, might include relaxation techniques and anxiety management to help reduce stress, which is possibly the most often cited reason for self-injury. A social skills group may consider allowing the individual to discover the effect he or she has on the environment in which they live. Creative groups such as art, drama and creative writing provide alternative ways of expressing and exploring feelings and emotions. Here we could use the experience of working with Ian as the example.

Case example

Ian was an 18-year-old man admitted to a low secure unit following a conviction for grievous bodily harm and sentencing to a young offenders unit where he regularly self-injured. He had a history of family separation, being taken into care and of both physical and sexual abuse. The diagnosis given was borderline personality disorder with unexplained but possibly drug-induced psychotic episodes. His attitude was 'I'm tough, you're not going to get near me and I'm not going to talk about it'. It was noted that instances of self-injury often followed angry outbursts, suggesting that release of stress or tension could be the reason. He refused to take part in the relaxation group saying that it was for wimps, but he was persuaded to try the musical ripple bed. This he admitted he enjoyed, and it was then that the occupational therapist was able to follow up with one-to-one sessions for him to learn other relaxation techniques. He was never persuaded to attend the relaxation group but did undertake one-to-one sessions for anxiety management as long as none of his peers knew what he was doing! It was during one of these sessions that it was explained that anger could precipitate self-injury. This came as a great revelation to him. It was also acceptable to his sense of pride. Sadly, although Ian is now living in the community, this was the only success, and, at present, he is deeply involved in drug misuse.

Longer-term interventions of assertiveness training, anger management, problem-solving and communication skills can all contribute to the building of self-confidence needed in returning to the community. Successful rehabilitation into the community has proved difficult for many forensic clients. They have to overcome the stigma not only of mental illness but also of being a lawbreaker. To explore this further the case of Sharon is a typical example of what might happen when the client is discharged.

Case example

When Sharon was about to be discharged from a secure unit, she was brought to the attention of the forensic outreach team via her Care Programme Approach Review and Mental Health Act (1983) Section 117 meeting. This team was then able to provide a continuing service to Sharon following her discharge. Sharon suffered from depression, possibly a result of a severely disturbed childhood, and prior to her admission to the low secure unit she had made two serious suicide attempts. She also had a history of self-injury at times of stress. The in-patient occupational therapy interventions had included self-esteem building, relaxation, anxiety management and assertiveness training. Sharon's expressed priority was to find employment, as 'worker' had been the only role in which she had experienced success in the past. Her greatest difficulties were in the area of social interaction and personal relationships. Because she had not been in employment for several years, Sharon decided that it would be useful to do some part-time voluntary work as a first step back on to the employment ladder. She became a general helper in a local charity shop where her eagerness to work was appreciated, and she soon became a valued asset. She also undertook a computer course at the local education centre, to provide her with a qualification as well as the opportunity to meet new people in an unforced way. This programme started to provide Sharon with both a structure to her life as well as roles. However, paid employment has proved elusive, even in an area of full employment. And following a number of rejections, she stopped applying. Leisure activities were also difficult to arrange for two reasons: first, because she was living on benefits she did not have much money to spend and, second, her social interaction skills were poor. She also did not want to attend activities specifically for people with mental health difficulties, because she felt that she needed to put that part of her life behind her. Her social life now revolves around her elderly neighbour with whom she has struck up a friendship, and occasional trips with one of the other helpers from the shop to the Ramblers Association.

It is unlikely that occupational therapists working within a forensic setting treat only patients who self-injure, but it may be possible to provide some group work that is specific to this client group. This may be a group that explores the individual's reasons for self-injury or one that accepts self-injury as a part of the individual's persona and concentrates on giving the knowledge to self-injure more safely. It is usual for these groups to be single gender, at least to begin with, but where it is possible to combine the groups at a later stage it can be useful, particularly to women, to discover their shared experiences. Even with the advent of organizations such as Childline, which has done so much to bring into the open the issue of child sexual abuse, many people believe that it is only girls who are abused and self-injure. The sharing of this experience can help women to break down some of the distrust of men per se, and for men to have their account accepted. These integrated groups must be allowed to happen only when the individual is emotionally ready, as forcing the issue will become self-defeating.

Conclusion

Anyone who works in a forensic setting will encounter patients or clients who self-injure. The reasons for needing to use this extreme coping mechanism can be many and varied but, whatever its cause, it is understanding, and not condemnation, that is required from the health professional. Working with people in such emotional pain is difficult and progress is slow, with many backward steps. Support is essential, and necessary for both patient and therapist while different strategies are tried. 'You can't go from A to Z overnight. Consider damage-limitation strategies in combination with *understanding* the reasons' (Pembroke 1994 p.56, italics added). It may be that a reduction in the injuries, together with education in the care of wounds, will be the outcome of the interventions, but one of the benefits clients have in forensic mental health settings is time. The length of stay for most forensic patients is usually greater than for most clients in either mental or physical health. This allows greater opportunity for long-term treatments. It is true, at the moment, that evidence for the inclusion of occupational therapy in the treatment of individuals who self-injure is of an anecdotal and impressionistic nature, but greater research could provide the evidence base for this work. Our core skills and holistic approach do appear to identify a role for occupational therapy, particularly in a forensic setting, to help in the relief from these overwhelming emotions.

References

Arnold L and Babiker G (1998) Counselling people who self-injure. In: Good Practice in Counselling People Who Have Been Abused, Bear Z (ed.). London: Jessica Kingsley.

Favazza A (1989) Why patients mutilate themselves. Hospital and Community Psychiatry 40(2) 137–145.

Favazza A and Conterio K (1989) Female habitual self-mutilators. Acta Psychiata Scand 79: 283–289.

Garner R, Butler G and Hutchings D (1994) A study of the relationship between the patterns of planned activity and incidents of deliberate self-harm within a regional secure unit. British Journal of Occupational Therapy 59(4) 156–160.

Haines J, Williams C and Brain K (1995) The psychopathology of incarcerated self-mutilators. Canadian Journal of Psychiatry 40(9) 514–522.

Hemkendreis M (1992) Increase in self-injuries on an inpatient psychiatric unit during evening hours. Hospital and Community Psychiatry 43(4) 394–395.

Levi M (1998) Basic Notes in Psychiatry (2nd edition). Reading: Petroc Press.

Pembroke L (ed.) (1994) Self-Harm: Perspectives from Personal Experience. London: Survivors Speak Out.

Tantam D and Whittaker J (1992) Personality disorder and self-wounding. British Journal of Psychiatry 161: 451–464.

Walsh M (2000) Deliberate Self-Harm – a retrospective overview of contagion behaviour amongst intensive care female patients in a British Special Hospital. Unpublished MSc thesis.

CHAPTER 18

Forensic addictive behaviours

JOHN CHACKSFIELD

Introduction

Possibly the least understood yet most problematic of issues affecting mentally disordered offenders and their offending is the issue of substance misuse and addictive behaviours. Addictive behaviours include any habit-forming behaviour, classically the use of illegal drugs or alcohol, and, where linked to offending, they are termed 'forensic addictive behaviours' (McKeown et al. 1996).

Alcohol and drug use has been associated with violence throughout history and examples of violent individuals such as Alexander the Great, Ivan the Terrible, Hitler, Stalin and even Henry VIII are cited frequently in the literature. Serial killers Geoffrey Dahmer and Dennis Nilsen were known to be alcoholics as well as having histories of violence (Graham 1996). Considerable evidence exists to suggest that drug misuse makes a significant contribution to the overall total of crimes committed in England and Wales in general (Hough 1995), and the correlation between alcohol or illicit substance misuse and crime is well established (Forshaw and Strang 1993, Hodge 1993, Goldstein 1989).

An increasing body of evidence has revealed that the use of alcohol and/or the use of drugs makes the clinical picture of any mental health client much more complicated. Commonly termed 'dual diagnosis', these issues are discussed in detail in the recent Government *Mental Health Policy Implementation Guide* on dual diagnosis (Department of Health 2002). The combination of mental illness and substance misuse becomes additionally complex when associated with criminal offending and more so when this leads to violence and murder.

Occupational therapists will encounter mentally disordered offenders who are also substance misusers or substance dependent in all levels of security. What will be most noticeable in these cases is the complexity of their needs and the significance of the effect on occupational performance. In addition, these clients are likely to take a considerable length of time to progress through the rehabilitation process and often present a poor prognosis on discharge (Chacksfield 2002). This chapter explores the impact of forensic addictive behaviours on occupational performance, the role that occupational therapists can play and strategies they can use as part of intervention and evaluation. The Model of Human Occupation is used to frame intervention (Kielhofner 1995, Kielhofner 2002).

The relationship between offending, addictive behaviour and mental disorder

More than a third of the high secure hospital population in 1992 suffered from alcohol-related problems and 7% were diagnosed with severe alcohol dependence as well as a major mental disorder (Quayle and Clarke 1992). One in ten male prisoners and one in four female prisoners in the same year were known to be using drugs (Reed 1992). More recent statistics have shown alcohol and drug use to be strongly associated with homicide (Appleby 2002). A significant research study providing evidence for the link between drug use and violence was the Epidemiological Catchment Area Survey (Swanson et al. 1990). This revealed that subjects from a large American sample who were diagnosed with both schizophrenia and substance misuse were three times more likely to report violence to others than those who were diagnosed with schizophrenia but not using substances.

The evidence for the link between offending and addictive behaviours that are not alcohol- or illicit-substance-related is less clear. Fazel et al. (1997) describe two cases with a dual diagnosis of pathological gambling and schizophrenia. In both cases, the high of the gambling was perceived as reducing the distress arising from their illness but the low felt on losing led to deterioration in their mental states. This in turn increased their drive to gamble. Both patients committed acquisitive offences to fund their habit, but in the process of committing these offences committed much more severe offences. One patient committed rape and the other homicide. Addiction has been linked to violence (Hodge 1997), sexual offending (McGregor and Howells 1997), joy riding (Kilpatrick 1997) and shoplifting (McGuire 1997). Brown (1997) hypothesizes that some forms of criminal offending are similar to some addictions. He relates this to the arousal levels that addictive behaviour can generate and how the behaviour is used to modulate arousal levels.

What is clear is that the many different forms of addictive behaviour, and behaviours that fit addiction models, will lead to complex needs in the clients. Much of the literature suggests that as addictive behaviour develops and increases in severity so does offending behaviour, and this is particularly problematic when a mental disorder is also present. Chacksfield and Forshaw (1997) present a diagram to represent the tripartite relationship between offending behaviour, addiction and mental disorder:

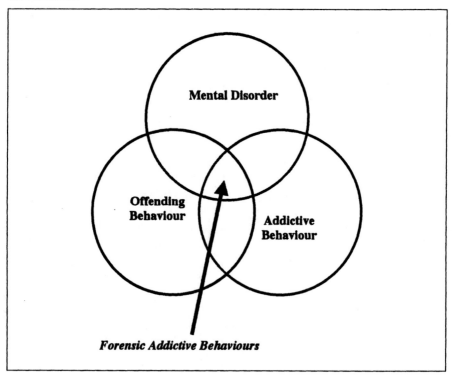

Figure 18.1 Diagram to represent the combination of mental disorder, offending behaviour and addictive behaviour known as 'forensic addictive behaviours' (Chacksfield and Forshaw 1997).

What is addictive behaviour?

Addictive behaviour is any behaviour that has the potential to become addictive. It is primarily linked to the use of alcohol or illicit substances. Four related concepts used here include:

1. **Substance misuse/problem use** refers to the use of alcohol or an illicit substance leading to the development of significant physical, mental or social problems.
2. **Substance dependence** refers to what is commonly called 'addiction' or 'dependence' as defined by the Dependence Syndrome in the *Diagnostic and Statistical Manual* (DSM IVR) (American Psychiatric Association 2000) and the International Classification of Disease (ICD-10) (World Health Organization 1992).

3. **Behavioural addiction** refers to non-substance-related addictive behaviours that have become pathological, such as gambling or some forms of repetitive sexual offending or violence.
4. **Dual diagnosis** has been defined as a broad spectrum of mental health and substance misuse problems that an individual might experience concurrently (Department of Health 2002). The nature of the relationship between these two conditions is complex. Possible mechanisms include:
   - a primary psychiatric illness precipitating or leading to substance misuse
   - substance misuse worsening or altering the course of a psychiatric illness
   - intoxication and/or substance dependence leading to psychological symptoms
   - substance misuse and/or withdrawal leading to psychiatric symptoms or illnesses.

The impact on occupational behaviour

The importance of occupational therapy and what makes its approach different from other healthcare practitioners is the emphasis on understanding the way pathology manifests in relation to occupational behaviour. Most theories surrounding addictive behaviours and mental disorder focus on the internal performance capacity element. The focus of occupational therapy is generally on the area of occupational performance.

As an example of the impact of forensic addictive behaviours on occupation, the case of Alfred is presented. Key aspects of his occupational lifestyle and how this developed are examined, as are the impact together with the natural history of his illness.

Case study

Alfred, a 28-year-old man, has been admitted to a maximum secure unit under Sections 37/41. His index offence was rape. He has a history of violent offending. His diagnosis on admission was schizophrenia, substance dependence and gambling addiction. At the age of 18 he began to exhibit the symptoms of paranoid schizophrenia, including auditory and visual hallucinations plus delusions with a sexual and religious content. At the same time he had an increasing dependence on cannabis, alcohol and gambling. He was 25 when he first used crack cocaine followed by intermittent but increased use over time. Alfred likes using these substances because, he says, they make him feel like a king, and he enjoys the social aspect of using drugs with friends.

Occupational lifestyle

Alfred's occupational lifestyle centred on social acceptability in his young adulthood. His parents had split up when he was 15, at which time he left school with no qualifications. Alfred was frequently beaten by his father and paternal grandmother, as were his brother and three step-siblings.

a) Family network: He lived with his mother who is alcohol dependent and sometimes with his paternal grandmother. His father saw him occasionally but mainly in the context of a betting shop. Alfred became well known within this context to several other male and female friends of his father.

b) Social network, axis 1 – betting shop: The betting shop experience was formative in Alfred's development. His father and other men developed betting 'systems' and Alfred became focused on developing the ideal winning system that would earn him money through betting on horses. This group tended to drink alcohol during and after betting sessions, then in the evenings while watching pornographic videos.

c) Social network, axis 2 – school and neighbourhood friends: Alfred stayed in contact with his childhood and school friends, particularly those who, like himself, were unemployed and on benefits and especially those who had entered a drug-using lifestyle. Over time, Alfred extended his social contacts through the drug-using subculture that he was becoming involved with. His criminal offending commenced within this group, with his need to pay for drugs.

Forensic history

Alfred's engagement in forensic occupations commenced with handbag snatching. Arrested on five occasions, he received convictions for petty theft, burglary, actual and grievous bodily harm. In addition he has served a custodial sentence for illegal possession of class A drugs and possession with intent to supply. Following two recent burglaries, he was convicted of indecent assault and rape. His index offence involved rape of an elderly woman.

Analysis of performance areas

a) Productivity (goal-directed activity aimed at financial reward): Alfred's main methods of obtaining the means to use drugs and to fund his activities are drug dealing and burglary. The drug dealing follows a pattern similar to regular employment in that Alfred operates a schedule of obtaining illegal drugs to supply to a list of customers with whom he maintains contact via his mobile phone. The burglary is less regular and follows a pattern similar to casual labour. Here Alfred commits burglary in order to obtain a fresh income when other sources have failed. With both of these occupations, Alfred's motivation comes from his drug habit, gambling habit and his need for social acceptance.

b) Leisure (activity aimed at relaxation and done for intrinsic reward): Alfred's main leisure activities centre on gambling in the betting shop, drinking alcohol and using drugs with friends. He spends a large amount of time in 'Shabeens' (illegal drinking venues), late-opening bars and at friends' houses.

c) Self-care: Alfred eats either at his mother's and grandmother's homes or eats takeaways. His diet is poor, and he does not cook for himself. He relies on his mother or grandmother to wash his clothes. His personal hygiene is generally poor and becomes better or worse in relation to his illness.

Alfred will require considerable assessment to identify the multiple elements of diagnosis. He clearly has a complex set of problems linked to the combination of addictive behaviour, mental illness and offending behaviour. Intervention will need to be multi-modal and multidisciplinary. The occupational therapist's contribution will focus on the impact of these problems on occupation.

Intervention and rehabilitation

The advantage that occupational therapists have with patients with complex needs is the holistic view that they take of a person's occupation, despite diagnosis or complexity. Three key steps are significant with patients with forensic addictive behaviours.

Engagement

Clinical experience shows that engagement with these clients occurs effectively through the medium of occupation. Commencing with engagement in non-threatening activities, such as art and crafts, trust can be built between therapist and client leading to a greater participation in group therapies.

An example of a successful artistic activity used with forensic addictive behaviour patients in maximum security is the use of a mural project to build self-esteem, self-efficacy and group interaction. In addition, the task enabled the group members to make choices about, and alter, the ward environment in which they lived. For each mural, a small group of three to five patients worked with the occupational therapist. The project involved joint planning, agreement of ideas, group motivation and sharing of equipment to achieve the desired result. The activity was designed to increase patients' self-efficacy and self-esteem by enabling them to successfully carry out a seemingly difficult task. For each mural, patients copied a picture from a book on to an overhead projector slide. The sketch was then projected on to a blank wall in a selected area of the ward and the outline used to transfer the picture on to the wall. This was then painted. The resulting effect, a near-perfect copy of the original, made all members of the group feel positive and pleased with their achievement. The additional benefit of being able to alter the ward environment, in a setting where there is considerable deprivation of choice, was significant in empowering the patients in the group. The activity was not directly psychotherapeutic or interpretative and was therefore perceived as non-threatening to the patients. This meant that the therapeutic goals of increasing self-esteem, group interaction and achievement could be met with little opposition. The therapist developed rapport and trust with the patients. The activity additionally prepared them for further group work, including more formal psychotherapeutic group sessions.

At this early stage the client may not be interested in focusing on issues relating to substance misuse or the problems that schizophrenia and other factors have caused in their lives. Yet once the client is engaged and trust has been built up between the client and the therapist, it is possible to move towards treatment strategies. For example, the Model of Change (Prochaska and DiClemente 1986) can be utilized to assist in formulating volitional strategies (Chacksfield and Lancaster 2002). This is a counselling model that structures intervention via five stages, namely: pre-contemplation, contemplation, determination, action, and maintenance. A sixth stage can be considered as relapse, where the person relapses to substance misuse and re-enters the cycle of change described. The value of this approach is that it clarifies that certain interventions will work only at certain stages of change. With occupational therapy, basic occupational engagement is appropriate at the early pre-contemplation stage, then later the patient can progress into occupations that are more focused on addressing specific issues around substance misuse, mental illness and offending.

Motivation

A key factor in establishing motivation is the development of self-esteem in the client. This can be facilitated through the direct use of purposeful occupation. As self-esteem grows, so does motivation. Close examination of the volitional sub-system (Kielhofner 1995) will assist the therapist to develop their reasoning in these areas. Clearly, substance users are motivated to use substances, and one aspect of intervention is to change or adapt this motivation to a less harmful form. Often clients will have had very minimal life experience of positive motivational situations. The majority of their volitional sub-system will have developed through negative experience or experience centred on drug misuse and criminal behaviour.

Key benefits of occupation occur when the client is able to take the small achievements obtained in occupational activity and generalize these to illness, offending or substance-misuse-related behaviour. Later stages of intervention will focus on these aspects via role playing and other group techniques as well as behavioural 'try-outs' where new skills can be rehearsed and practised in occupation-based sessions.

An example from practice is where a patient identifies that experiencing social conflict can act as a trigger to relapse. In a social skills session they may learn strategies to be assertive and to handle conflict without resorting to violence or substance misuse. Additionally they may learn about assertiveness and handling conflict without resorting to violence. They may need help to transfer these skills to a realistic, occupation-based setting. In a high secure setting, in the bricklayers department this occurred where patients had to work as a team to achieve a building task. Interpersonal conflict could occur in these settings; however, it may be orchestrated in a safe way, for example by encouraging patients to change roles within the bricklaying team from participant to leader.

Additional triggers to relapse may come from the environment itself, particularly where a client plans to return to their old substance-using locations. A clear example is the return to social activities in pubs. Here the environment can 'press' (Kielhofner 1995) or support certain behaviours, including relapse to alcohol use. The sight of a bar or the smell of alcohol can trigger a desire to drink alcohol. Occupational therapy can assist the development of strategies to reduce response to these triggers.

Within a forensic addictive behaviours unit in a high secure setting the occupational therapist set up a mock bar environment to assist patients with alcohol problems to rehearse assertiveness strategies and cope with a pub environment. The 'bar session' included five patients each diagnosed with alcohol dependence. The bar was set up so that one patient was the customer, purchasing an alcoholic drink. Behind the bar were four patients plus the therapist as bar staff. The goal of the bar staff was to persuade the customer to buy a drink in as many ways as possible. The goal of the customer was to resist in as many ways as possible. The group members rotated so that each member could perform in each role. The therapist was included in this in order to model drink-refusing tactics and responses. Patients responded well to this activity, and it was carried out as part of a social skills programme, including assertion training and stress management. The value of role playing was significant in helping patients think about relapse prevention strategies.

Occupational balance

A primary concern with return to community living for these clients is the ability to establish and maintain a balanced occupational lifestyle. This needs to consist of a sustained and equal balance of productivity, leisure and self-care. Within the hospital, they are provided with an artificial, institutional structure that forces a specific pattern of occupation. On discharge, major problems can occur when the structure that they have become used to ceases to exist. A graded re-entry to community living is therefore essential. This includes group work that looks at pre-discharge issues, in particular encouragement to explore environmental or occupational triggers to relapse and identifying strategies for managing or coping with these. Carrying these out with a strong occupational focus is particularly effective in reconstructing the habituation sub-system within the client and ensuring a successful return to community life.

Occupational therapists at the Bracton Centre, a medium secure setting, have made use of two types of groups to facilitate the client's development of occupational balance. These groups are led by the occupational therapist and supported by nursing staff. One group is the Substance Use and Awareness Group. This is primarily an information and education-based group that aims to assist clients in understanding the role that drugs and alcohol may have played in their illness and offending behaviour. The expected outcome of the group is that clients will have a greater understanding and knowledge of many aspects of substance misuse. It may also support them to begin to consider relapse prevention. The second group is the Stopping Substances Group. This group reintroduces the idea of relapse prevention. The group follows a structure that aims to develop participants' motivation to change their patterns of substance use and to learn strategies and techniques to help change substance misuse behaviour and prevent relapse in the community. The group emphasizes the need to appreciate each individual's readiness to change their behaviour and to tailor the approach made within the group to individual needs.

Case Study

Marshall is a 30-year-old man who has been diagnosed with paranoid schizophrenia and problem drug use. His main drug of choice is cannabis. Marshall was referred to the Substance Use and Awareness Group in order to increase his awareness about cannabis and its effects on his mental state. During the group he learnt:

* about the effect of cannabis on his mental state
* facts about cannabis, its classification and legal status
* facts about legal penalties in relation to cannabis.

As a member of the group, Marshall was able to listen to others' experiences of harder drug use, which deterred him from progressing to using these substances. His self-awareness improved in relation to situations that he identified as triggers to cannabis use. He then developed strategies he could use to deter himself. Here the facilitators introduced some initial ideas around relapse prevention. Finally, the group introduced Marshall to the types of services available within the community that would support him in changing his patterns of substance use.

These kinds of group interventions can be highly successful when coupled with opportunities for rehearsal within an occupational environment and run in conjunction with a multidisciplinary relapse prevention initiative.

Individual sessions are also important in supporting occupational change and planning for return to community life. In this, a primary value is the transmission to the patient of a vision of life 'as it will be'. Using theory from Solution Focused Therapy (see Miller and Berg 1997) can assist the development of a positive occupational vision. Many patients tend to focus on 'the discharge date' as the end-point of treatment and therefore the focus of intervention, for them, is related to this goal. The importance of occupational therapy is in assisting the development of a vision of a positive lifestyle in the community away from potential relapse situations. This is particularly important for patients with forensic addictive behaviours, as they have a multiplicity of potential relapse opportunities.

Evaluation and outcome measurement

It is recommended that standard occupational therapy measurement materials are used, such as the Volitional Questionnaire (De las Heras et al. 1998), the Occupational Performance History Interview (Version II)

(Kielhofner et al. 2001) and the Occupational Self-Assessment (OSA) (Baron et al. 2002). These assessments have been subject to rigorous development and testing for reliability and validity. New assessments and the latest references for these are available online at the Model of Human Occupation Clearing House website (http://www.uic.edu/ahp/OT/ MOHOC/).

In addition, they focus on occupational performance and are sensitive to change. For measurement of cognition, self-perception, self-esteem and coping, there is a range of instruments available via the psychology literature. However, these are not occupational performance-based instruments, and, although they can contribute to reasoning and clinical judgement, they do not ultimately measure changes in occupational behaviour. Wherever possible, clients should be involved in assessment and reassessment as part of the ongoing volitional engagement process. Additional evaluation will occur through team meetings and individual sessions with the client where treatment objectives are revisited and developed further.

Conclusion

The issues presented by the combination of mental disorder, substance misuse and offending behaviour are considerable in their impact on occupation. Occupational therapy has a key role to play in addressing a return to a balanced lifestyle that does not involve relapse to these three interacting areas of behaviour. In particular, occupational therapists can assist patients to increase their engagement in treatment through stages, increasing the development of self-esteem, skills for coping and lifestyle management over time. Rehearsal of these skills through occupational activity can assist in the return to successful living in the community and prevention of relapse to illness and substance misuse leading to re-offending.

References

American Psychiatric Association (2000) Diagnostic and Statistical Manual of Mental Disorders (4th edition) (DSM IVR). Washington: American Psychiatric Publishing.

Appleby L (2002) Safety First: Five-year Report of the National Confidential Enquiry into Suicides and Homicide by People with Mental Illness. London: Department of Health.

Baron K, Kielhofner G, Iyenger A, Goldhammer V and Wolenski J (2002) The Occupational Self-Assessment Version 2.0. Chicago: University of Illinois.

Brown I (1997) A theoretical model of the behavioural addictions – applied to offending. In: Addicted to Crime? Hodge J, McMurran M and Hollin C (eds.). Chichester: Wiley.

Chacksfield J and Forshaw D (1997) Occupational therapy and forensic addictive behaviours. British Journal of Therapy and Rehabilitation 4(7) 381–386.

Chacksfield J and Lancaster J (2002) Substance misuse. In: Occupational Therapy and Mental Health (3rd edition), Creek J (ed.). Edinburgh: Churchill Livingstone.

Chacksfield J (2002) Rehabilitation: the long haul. In: All Drink, Drugs and Dependence: From Science to Clinical Practice, Caan W and DeBelleroche J (eds.). London: Butterworth Heinemann.

Department of Health (2002) Mental Health Policy Implementation Guide: Dual Diagnosis Good Practice Guide. London: Department of Health.

De las Heras C, Geist R and Kielhofner G (1998) Manual for the Volitional Questionnaire. Chicago: Model of Human Occupation Clearing House

Fazel S, Chapman M and Forshaw D (1997) Pathological gambling and mental illness: a dangerous combination? Journal of Psychiatric Case Reports 2(1) 87–94.

Forshaw D and Strang J (1993) Drugs, aggression and violence. In: Violence in Society, Taylor P (ed.). London: Royal College of Physicians.

Graham J (1996) The Secret History of Alcoholism. Shaftesbury: Element.

Goldstein P (1989) Drugs and violent crime. In: Pathways to Criminal Violence, Weiner N and Wolfgang M (eds.). California: Sage.

Hodge J (1993) Alcohol and violence. In: Violence in Society, Taylor P (ed.). London: Royal College of Physicians.

Hodge J, McMurran M and Hollin C (1997) Introduction: Current issues in the treatment of addictions and crime. In: Addicted to Crime? Hodge J, McMurran M and Hollin C (eds.). Chichester: Wiley.

Hough M (1995) Drug Misuse and the Criminal Justice System: a review of the literature. London: Home Office Drugs Prevention Initiative.

Kielhofner G (ed.) (1995) Model of Human Occupation: Theory and Application (2nd edition). Baltimore: Williams and Wilkins.

Kielhofner G (ed.) (2002) Model of Human Occupation: Theory and Application (3rd edition). Baltimore: Lippincott Williams and Wilkins.

Kielhofner G, Mallinson T, Forsyth K and Lai J (2001) Psychometric properties of the second version of the Occupational Performance History Interview (OPHI-II). American Journal of Occupational Therapy 55(3) 260–267.

Kilpatrick R (1997) Joy-Riding: An addictive behaviour? In: Addicted to Crime? Hodge J, McMurran M and Hollin C (eds.). Chichester: Wiley.

McGregor G and Howells K (1997) Addiction models of sexual offending. In: Addicted to Crime? Hodge J, McMurran M and Hollin C (eds.). Chichester: Wiley.

McGuire J (1997) 'Irrational' shoplifting and models of addiction. In: Addicted to Crime? Hodge J, McMurran M and Hollin C (eds.). Chichester: Wiley.

McKeown O, Forshaw D, McGauley G, Fitzpatrick J and Roscoe J (1996) Forensic addictive behaviours unit: A case study (part 1). Journal of Substance Misuse 1(1) 27–31.

Miller S and Berg I (1997) The Miracle Method: A Radically New Approach to Problem Drinking. New York: WW Norton.

Prochaska J and DiClemente C (1986) Towards a comprehensive model of change. In: Treating Addictive Behaviours: Processes of Change, Miller RJ and Heather N (eds.). London: Plenum.

Quayle M and Clarke F (1992) Alcohol and Special Hospitals. Broadmoor Hospital: Internal Report (personal communication).

Reed J (1992) Review of Health and Social Services for Mentally Disordered Offenders and Others Requiring Similar Services, Volume 5: Special Issues. London: HMSO.

Swanson J, Holzer C, Ganju V and Jonu R (1990) Violence and psychiatric disorder in the community: Evidence from the epidemiological catchment area surveys. Hospital and Community Psychiatry 41(7) 761–770.

World Health Organization (1992) The ICD-10 Classification of Mental and Behavioural Disorders: Clinical Descriptions and Diagnostic Guidelines. Geneva: World Health Organization.

Acknowledgement

The author wishes to thank the professionals from the Bracton Centre medium secure unit for provision of the case example 'Marshall'.

CHAPTER 19

Occupational therapy and the sexual offender

EDWARD DUNCAN

Introduction

> If I can get through to a person, even those whose behaviour has a lot of destructive elements, I believe he or she would want to do the right thing.
> Carl Rogers.
>
> (quoted in Baldwin and Satir 1987 p.45)

Few crimes appear to elicit a stronger reaction from society than those of sexual offences. Sexual offenders are to be found in a variety of environments in which occupational therapists work: secure units/hospitals, prisons and community settings. Of those in institutions, the vast majority of sexual offenders are located in prison services. This is due to the fact that the overwhelming majority of such offenders are not diagnostically mentally ill. Paradoxically, it is probably occupational therapists, working in forensic hospitals, of varying levels of security, that have most contact with sexual offenders. Undoubtedly, this relates to the low number of occupational therapists currently employed by the prison service. The publication of *The Future Organisation and Delivery of Prison Health Care* (Health Service Circular 1999) will hopefully enable an increasing number of occupational therapists to work in this setting. Treating sexual offenders has been described as one of the most demanding tasks of a mental health professional (Blanchard 1998). This chapter provides the reader with an introduction to this challenging area.

To date, the role of occupational therapy with this client group has been largely undocumented. The chapter commences with a brief overview of the categorization of sexual offences, both diagnostic and legislative. The theoretical basis of sexual offending will then be explored. Following this, the role of the occupational therapist in this area will be discussed. Of all the challenges facing therapists working with this client group, the maintenance of a congruent therapeutic relationship is perhaps the most challenging. It is for this reason that the final section of the chapter is dedicated specifically to the therapeutic relationship.

Categorization of sexual offences

Sexual offences are classified in various ways. Both the legal system and the health sector classify sexual offences differently, according to their needs. This section outlines the classification criteria for both systems. Classification systems, by their nature, are arbitrary and include a degree of overlap. Each system differs in its focus: description of offence in relation to behaviour, by choice of victim or by presence of mental disorder (Prins 1995).

Healthcare classifications

Within both the *Diagnostic and Statistical Manual* (DSM IVR) and the *International Classification of Diseases* (ICD-10), sexual offences are termed 'paraphilias' and are listed in the chapter relating to Sexual and Gender Identity Disorders under section 302.00 DSM IVR (American Psychiatric Association 2000) and F65 (World Health Organization 1992). The term 'paraphilia' derives from the Greek words *para* 'beyond' and *philia* 'fondness for'.

The defining aspects of a paraphilic diagnosis are as follows:

- recurrent, intense sexually arousing fantasies, sexual urges or behaviours, which involve non-human objects, self-humiliation or humiliation of one's partner, children or a non-consenting person
- such behaviour must last for a period of at least six months
- the sexual urges, behaviour or fantasies must cause significant distress or impairment on social, occupational or other important areas of functioning.

Both the DSM IVR (American Psychiatric Association 2000) classification of sexual offences and the ICD-10 (World Health Organization 1992) classification differ in content, and the reader is referred to these texts for detailed information.

An interesting omission, which one might have expected to see, is the classification of rape, which does not exist in either of the diagnostic manuals. This is due to the fact that the offence is largely violence-based rather than aimed at achieving sexual satisfaction as its sole need (Prins 1995). In order to understand the offence of rape more clearly, it is necessary to consider a further classification system of this singular offence. Such a system is offered by Groth and Hobson (1983):

1. **anger rape** – motivated by feeling 'put down' or by retribution for perceived wrongs
2. **power rape** – engaged in as a means of denting deep feelings of inadequacy and insecurity
3. **sadistic rape** – victims are usually complete strangers; they may be subjected to torture, bondage and highly deviant sexual practices.

This classification system is not comprehensive and has been criticized by others. A more detailed classification of those who commit rape is provided by Prins (1995).

Legislative criteria

> Sexual offences constitute a very small proportion of all crimes, something in the order of 2% of all recorded offences and about 1.75% of all persons found guilty of indictable offences. There is also a discrepancy between the numbers of sexual offences known to the police and the number actually dealt with or prosecuted ... in addition, many more offences are committed than are ever reported to the police.
>
> (Prins 1995 p.201)

Sexual offences can be classified under a variety of legislature. Some of these are not immediately recognizable as being related to sexual offending (e.g. breach of the peace). Key acts of parliament directly relating to sexual offending include: Sex Offences Act (1956) and the Sex Offenders Act (1997). The Sex Offenders Act (1997) has been amended within the Criminal Justice and Court Services Act (2000). These amendments relate to the initial registration of sexual offenders with police.

Theoretical basis of sexual offending

Despite several years of examining the issues surrounding sexual offending, the origins of sexual assault remain unclear (Marshall et al. 1990). A proliferation of theories exist which attempt to explain sexual assault, ranging from sociological concepts to micro theories, aetiological constructs to maintaining factors. It has been stated that 'all human behaviour is multiply determined by a complex of many interacting variables' (Marshall et al. 1990 p.6), and the array of theoretical development which has occurred within sexual offending appears to validate this position. Several publications exist which detail the theoretical basis of sexual offending (Clark and Erooga 1994, Marshall et al. 1990, Ward and Hudson 1998). Despite the wealth of literature in the area, there continues to be an absence of an integrated theory that could provide a global rationale for the onset, development and maintenance of sexual offending (Ward and Hudson 1998).

Occupational therapy interventions

The assessment and treatment of sex offenders by occupational therapists is an area of human behaviour that is filled with unique problems and *has not been well studied*.

(Lloyd 1987 p.55, emphasis added).

It is with a degree of frustration that the above statement, quoted from the sole article pertaining to occupational therapy and sex offenders, is as true today as it was 15 years ago. Despite the increase in occupational therapists working in secure settings (Duncan 1999a), little remains published regarding sexual offenders. The rationale for this may be manifold:

- Occupational therapy in forensic care is itself a developing speciality (Chacksfield 1997). Therefore, the focus of publications, to date, has been on role definition in the area.
- The field of sexual offender rehabilitation is one that many professionals find unattractive to work in and are overcome with personal feelings regarding the individual and their offence(s).
- As few occupational therapists are located in prisons, where occupational therapists could have a high degree of contact with sex offenders, there has been less opportunity for research.
- Occupational therapy interventions with sexual offenders may not differ significantly from interventions with other forensic patient populations.

It is most likely that a combination of the above reasons, and perhaps others not listed, have led to a dearth of literature in this area. This section outlines the current role of occupational therapists working with sexual offenders. Owing to the lack of research, the recommendations given are drawn from the sole publication to date on the topic (Lloyd 1987), relevant information from multidisciplinary publications, and clinical experience in the field.

A variety of interventions

Marshall (1996), a psychologist internationally recognized for his clinical and research expertise in sexual offending, divides the treatment of sexual offenders into two categories: offence-related and offence-specific (Table 19.1). The distinction of these two categories does not imply that some areas are more important than others. Instead, it clarifies those areas that always require intervention (offence-specific) compared with other areas (offence-related), which may not be relevant to all sexual offenders. A systematic review of the management of sexual offenders has been published by the Cochrane Collaboration (White et al. 2001).

In Great Britain, a programme of sexual offender rehabilitation, focusing upon offence-specific interventions, has been developed within the prison service. The sexual offender treatment programme (SOTP) has been widely implemented throughout the country, and variations of the programme have been developed for individuals with learning difficulties and mentally disordered offenders. These programmes focus upon the offence-specific aspects of interventions. While occupational therapists have become involved in the delivery of SOTP interventions, it should be recognized that their involvement as an occupational therapist is at the level of shared skill (Duncan 1999b). More important for the future development of occupational therapy and sexual offender rehabilitation is the occupational therapist's interventions at the level of offence-related interventions. Lloyd (1987 p.62) states that 'a major goal of occupational therapy, underlying all other treatment goals is to increase the sex offender's appraisal skills so that he is able to identify his own strengths, weaknesses and needs ... The focus on treatment of the sex offender is on maximizing the potential of the individual to cope with non-deviant life experiences.' It is in this arena that the occupational therapist's core skills (Duncan 1999a) can be utilized to their full potential.

Table 19.1 Categories of interventions for sexual offenders

Offence-specific interventions	Offence-related interventions
Denial/minimization	Relationship/marital therapy
Victim harm/empathy	Anger management
Offence-supportive attitudes	Substance abuse awareness
Beliefs and disordered perceptions	Social skills and assertiveness training
Offence fantasies	Life-management skills
Relapse prevention	

The occupational therapist as part of a multidisciplinary team

Multidisciplinary working is essential when an occupational therapist is involved in working with sexual offenders because:

- Working with sexual offenders can be very stressful. Working as part of a team enables support and consultancy from other colleagues who are aware of the patient's history.

- It assists in the development of adequate resources, both practical and professional, for working with this group (for example group room space, supervision, leadership, etc.)
- It ensures that interventions are provided to individuals at appropriate points in their rehabilitation. One important example of this is social skill interventions, 'it is important to ensure that provision of social skills training is not based on a misapprehension from sexual offending. Without increasing victim awareness and empathy, enhancement of social skills for this client group can present the risk of developing a more socially skilled offender' (Clark and Erooga 1994 p. 114). The development of effective communication skills may well be an appropriate occupational therapy goal. However, the timing of such an intervention, within the individual's overall rehabilitation, is of importance.

Clinical approaches and models of practice

In the author's clinical practice, two approaches, or models, are utilized in occupational therapy interventions with sexual offenders: the cognitive behavioural approach and the Model of Human Occupation (Kielhofner 2002).

The cognitive behavioural approach

The majority of sexual offender programmes of rehabilitation utilize a cognitive behavioural approach (Beckett 1994). This approach is appropriate for both offence-specific interventions as well as the offence-related interventions. Occupational therapists frequently use this approach for skills-acquisition training. It can also be effectively utilized to develop levels of self-esteem, a construct known to be lacking among sex offenders, particularly paedophiles (Fisher 1994). The utilization of a cognitive behavioural approach by occupational therapists is not without its critics, who suggest that it creates a blurring of roles and leads to a loss of professional identity. Such criticism should be balanced against the overwhelming evidence base for cognitive behavioural interventions in a variety of settings and its inherent interdisciplinary nature. A fuller discussion of the practice of the cognitive behavioural approach by occupational therapists can be found in Duncan (in press).

The Model of Human Occupation

Currently, within Great Britain, occupational therapists working in secure settings are increasingly adopting the Model of Human Occupation (MoHO) as their core occupational therapy model for practice. There are several reasons for this:

- Clinical governance demands that occupational therapists utilize the best possible level of evidence base to support their interventions. The Model of Human Occupation is probably the most comprehensive occupational therapy model, with over 20 years of development – both theoretical and practical.
- The model's definitions of volition, habituation and performance are of direct relevance to sexual offender rehabilitation:

  1. Volition – The understanding of sexual offenders' motivation to offend is complex. The occupational therapist's role is to assist in the development of volition to participate in activities which are congruent with the individual's level of occupational performance and are pro-social.
  2. Habituation – Many sexual offenders will have poorly developed 'habits', and a 'role' of offender. In these situations, the occupational therapist should work with the individual to develop pro-social habits and the formation of a variety of roles that support a non-offending future. This is important as sexual offenders need to 'get positive rewards in what they are normally doing so they do not have to resort to sexual assault as a reward or as a way of feeling adequate' (Lloyd 1987).
  3. Performance – Sexual offenders frequently present with performance-skill deficits. Social-competency deficits among sexual offenders have been well documented (Marshall 1996, McFall 1990). It is also recognized that these individuals will often have poorly developed performance in life skills (Lloyd 1987, Marshall 1996).

- MoHO has developed several assessments, and assessments have been developed closely based upon the model. These assessments provide various manners of information gathering and outcome measurement: interview, self-report and observation. These methods present challenges for the therapist when working with sexual offenders:

  1. Interview: *The Occupational Performance History Interview II* (OPHI II) (Kielhofner et al. 2001) provides a comprehensive overview of an individual's occupational performance, from an historical perspective. The interview provides an opportunity to develop rapport with the individual and to begin to socialize the client to the role of the occupational therapist. As sexual offenders frequently deny and minimize their offence, it is important that the therapist is aware of the background information prior to the interview, in order not to unwittingly reinforce the individual's minimization or denial.

2. Self-Report: Several self-report measures exist within the MoHO. Perhaps the most relevant of these is the *Role Checklist* (Oakley et al. 1986). While such assessments are valuable and should be utilized when indicated, a word of caution should be added when utilizing them with sexual offenders. Sexual offenders are frequently cited as unreliable when self-reporting (Fisher 1994). While such poor self-reporting is mostly related to offence-specific aspects of assessment, clinical experience has also illustrated that sexual offenders are also frequently unreliable self-reporters when assessed on offence-related components.

3. Observational measures. Three excellent observational measures exist within the model, which can provide accurate and detailed information regarding sexual offenders' occupational performance. These are:

   - The *Assessment of Communication and Interaction Skills* (ACIS) (Forsyth et al. 1999) provides an assessment for examining the individual's levels of social competency in a variety of environments.
   - The *Assessment of Motor and Process Skills* (AMPS) (Baron 1994), the most developed of the three assessments, provides an accurate rating of the individual's motor and process skills. This information is essential in understanding the likelihood of successful community reintegration, of sexual offenders, from a life-skills perspective.
   - The *Volitional Questionnaire* (VQ) (Chern et al. 1996), a confusingly named assessment is in fact an observational measure and not a self-report instrument. The VQ allows for the individual's levels of volition to be measured in a variety of different environments and with varying degrees of interaction with other people. The VQ was specifically developed for lower-functioning individuals with enduring mental illness or learning difficulty and therefore may not always be sensitive to the volitional deficits of higher-functioning sexual offenders.

A third edition of the key text (Kielhofner 2002) has recently been published. Interested readers are directed to this text, and to the MoHO website (www.uic.edu/ahp/OT/MOHOC/), for the latest developments within the model. Until now, the use of the MoHO in relation to sexual offender rehabilitation has not been defined. It is vital, however, that the profession moves to studying the efficacy of the model and its applications with sexual offenders.

Engaging with sexual offenders

In the minds of most, sexual offenders are hideous monsters. Indeed, the Scots call them 'beasts' and all societies have their own colloquial derogatories for these offenders.

(Marshall 1996 p.162)

It would be remiss to conclude this chapter without addressing the reality of the personal and professional challenges facing occupational therapists that work with this client group. Many therapists, aware of their own perspectives of sexual offenders, state that they could not work with such individuals. Such a stance should be respected; it would hardly be a beneficial relationship, for either party, to enforce a therapeutic relationship. It should be recognized, however, that the prevalence of sexual offending is such that many occupational therapists will unwittingly already be working with sexual offenders. Perhaps such opinions are more influenced by myth and media than by reality. This section briefly discusses some of the issues of engaging with sexual offenders in a therapeutic relationship.

Difficult people

When we look beneath the surface, beneath the impulsive evil deed, we see within our enemy-neighbour a measure of goodness and know that the viciousness and evilness of his acts are not quite representative of all that he is. We see him in a new light.

(King 1963)

Offenders, and sexual offenders in particular, can often be difficult people to engage with. It is not uncommon, although unethical, to hear professionals of all disciplines referring to sexual offenders in degrading terms. There are several reasons for this:

- **Societal**: Society is repulsed by such offences, and, when sexual offences come to light, all levels of community unite in their 'disbelief and rage' at such events. Such feelings escalate when the offender is discovered to be a professional, respected community member, 'we like to believe that sex crimes are committed only by demented and perverted individuals living in distant places, not by people we know in our own communities' (Blanchard 1998 p.13).
- **Professional**: Sexual offenders often communicate (orally and non-verbally) with the therapist in an abrasive, manipulative and/or unpleasant manner. Such interactions are difficult and challenging for the therapist to cope with. Frequently, professionals appear tempted to

utilize self-protection strategies (such as ignoring the individuals) or limit setting (such as terminating the conversation, seeing the individual as little as possible) to cope with the situation. In place of these defensive strategies, the patient's method of communicating should be evaluated, instead of the content or the subjective responses of the therapist (Blanchard 1998). Frequently, such a presentation is indicative of underlying clinical difficulties. When framed in this manner, the difficult communication style of the individual can be reformulated and understood as an indication of his difficulties and occupational performance deficits.

- **Personal**: The offender's victim(s) may bear similarities in age, gender or other factors to a relative or friend of the therapist. Frequently, the offences of sexual offenders are reported in the local and national press, together with pictures and reports from the victims and their families. Such reports tend to be more personal in nature than the reports available in the individual's records. In one sense, this avoids the therapist splitting the offender from the crime, by reinforcing the nature and severity of the offence. Such experiences, however, can affect the therapeutic relationship and should be brought to clinical supervision.

The importance of supervision

Given the above discussion, clinical supervision should be given a central place in the timetable of the forensic occupational therapist. Clinical supervision should provide a supportive environment in which to discuss progress in each individual's therapeutic programme as well as the professional challenges of dealing with such individuals. Supervision should also be a safe place in which the supervisee can discuss any personal issues resulting from working with sexual offenders.

Summary

This chapter has reviewed the role of the occupational therapist when working with sexual offenders. The lack of research in the field has been noted and the importance of working as part of a multidisciplinary team reiterated. Two models of practice have been proposed as particularly useful when engaging in therapy. The personally challenging nature of working with sexual offenders has been highlighted. Such beliefs are often fuelled more by myth and perceived ideas of working with sexual offenders than by reality. Effective supervision is vital to provide a safe place to air such concerns and enable the effective practice of occupational therapy with sexual offenders. Much research needs to be carried out with this challenging population. A professional aspiration must be to make the next 15 years in this area more productive than the last.

References

American Psychiatric Association (2000) Diagnostic and Statistical Manual of Mental Disorders (4th edition) (DSM IVR). Washington DC: American Psychiatric Association.

Baldwin M and Satir V (eds.) (1987) The Use of Self in Therapy. Haworth: New York.

Baron K (1994) Clinical interpretation of 'The Assessment of Motor and Process Skills of Persons With Psychiatric Disorders' (AMPS). American Journal of Occupational Therapy 48(9) 781–782.

Beckett R (1994) Cognitive behavioural treatment of sex offenders. In: Sexual Offending Against Children: Assessment and Treatment of Male Abusers. Morrison T, Erooga M and Beckett R (eds.). London: Routledge.

Blanchard G (1998) The Difficult Connection: The Therapeutic Relationship in Sex Offender Treatment. Vermont: Safer Society Press.

Chacksfield J (1997) Forensic occupational therapy: Is it a developing specialism? British Journal of Therapy and Rehabilitation. Occupational Therapy Supplement of Forensic Psychiatry 4(7) 371–374.

Chern J, Kielhofner G, de las Heras C and Magalhaes L (1996) The Volitional Questionnaire (VQ): Psychometric development and practical use. American Journal of Occupational Therapy 50(7) 516–25.

Clark P and Erooga M (1994) Group work with men who sexually abuse children. In: Sexual Offending Against Children: Assessment and Treatment of Male Abusers. Morrison T, Erooga M and Beckett R (eds.). London: Routledge.

Criminal Justice and Court Services Act (2000) London: The Stationery Office.

Duncan E (1999a) Forensic services and occupational therapy: A developing area of practice? Occupational Therapy News 7(10) 24.

Duncan E (1999b) Occupational therapy in mental health: It is time to recognise that it has come of age. The British Journal of Occupational Therapy 62(11) 521–522.

Duncan E (in press) Cognitive behaviour therapy. In: Physiotherapy and Occupational Therapy in Mental Health: An Evidence-based Approach. Everett T, Donaghy M and Feaver S. London: Butterworth Heinemann.

Fisher D (1994) Adult sexual offenders: Who are they? What and how do they do it? In: Sexual Offending Against Children: Assessment and Treatment of Male Abusers. Morrison T, Erooga M and Beckett R (eds.). London: Routledge.

Forsyth K, Lai J and Kielhofner G (1999) The assessment of communication and interaction skills (ACIS): Measurement properties. British Journal of Occupational Therapy 62(2) 69–74.

Groth A and Hobson W (1983) The dynamics of sexual assault. In: Sexual Dynamics of Anti-social Behaviour. Schlesinger L and Revitch E (eds.). Ohio: Springsfield.

Health Service Circular (1999) The Future Organisation and Delivery of Prison Health Care. Health Service Circular 1999/077. London: Department of Health.

Kielhofner G (ed.) (2002) Model of Human Occupation: Theory and Application (3rd edition). Baltimore: Williams and Wilkins.

Kielhofner G, Mallinson T, Forsyth K and Lai J (2001) Psychometric properties of the second version of the Occupational Performance History Interview (OPHI-II). American Journal of Occupational Therapy 55(3) 260–267.

King M (1963) Strength to Love. Philadelphia: Fortress.

Lloyd C (1987) Sex offender programs: Is there a role for occupational therapy? Occupational Therapy in Mental Health 7(3) 55–67.

Marshall W (1996) Assessment, treatment and theorizing about sex offenders: Developments during the past twenty years and future directions. Criminal Justice and Behaviour 23(1) 162–199.

Marshall W, Laws D and Barbaree H (1990) Issues in sexual assault. In: Handbook of Sexual Assault: Issues, Theories and Treatment of the Offender, Marshall W, Laws D and Barbaree H (eds.). New York: Plenum.

McFall R (1990) The enhancement of social skills: An information-processing analysis. In: Handbook of Sexual Assault: Issues, Theories and Treatment of the Offender, Marshall W, Laws D and Barbaree H (eds.). New York: Plenum.

Oakley F, Kielhofner G, Barris R and Reichler D (1986) The role checklist: Development and empirical assessment of reliability. The Occupational Therapy Journal of Research 6(3) 57–161.

Prins H (1995) Offenders, Deviants or Patients (2nd edition). London: Routledge.

Sex Offences Act (1956) London: The Stationery Office.

Sex Offences (Amendment) Act (1976) London: The Stationery Office.

Sex Offenders Act (1997) London: The Stationery Office.

Ward T and Hudson S (1998) The construction and development of theory in the sexual offending area: A meta-theoretical framework. Sexual Abuse: A Journal of Research and Treatment (10)2 47–63.

White P, Bradley C, Ferriter M and Hatzipetrou L (2001) Managements for People with Disorders of Sexual Preference and for Convicted Sexual Offenders (Cochrane Review) The Cochrane Library Issue 4. Oxford: Update Software.

World Health Organization (1992) The ICD-10 Classification of Mental and Behavioural Disorders. Geneva: World Health Organization.

CHAPTER 20

Personality disorder – a role for occupational therapy

LORNA COULDRICK

Introduction

Every week the newspapers are filled with dramatic headlines arising from the behaviour of people deemed to have a personality disorder. Sometimes they are pejoratively labelled psychopaths and both fictional and non-fictional accounts of their notorious exploits fill the bookstalls. The very term engenders powerful emotions, from intrigue and fascination to disgust, revulsion and loathing but, above all else, it evokes divisions of opinion. This chapter briefly explores the controversy particularly surrounding the definition, diagnosis, causal factors and treatability of those with a personality disorder. It will attempt to move from tabloid headlines to an understanding of the issues, illustrated through personal experience, of working with people, detained in a medium secure unit under the Mental Health Act (1983), who are psychopathic.

Despite the dissent, one thing is certain; these people, wherever they are placed, engage in activity. Like all humans, they have an innate drive towards occupational behaviour. It is in understanding and using this, matching appropriate activity to the assessed need, that one defines occupational therapy. It is proposed that the core skills of occupational therapy are valuable in the management and treatment of people diagnosed with a personality disorder within both health and prison services. The tasks people engage in can become more than a way of passing time or managing behaviour. Activity can provide a framework to assess functional skills, social skills and intrapersonal understanding. It can be used to increase self-exploration and awareness. It can be structured to reinforce or develop patterns of behaviour and provide feedback. It can help individuals identify the need to change, and it can support rehearsal and practice in changing. Furthermore, establishing an appropriate balance of occupation can maintain individuals after release or discharge.

It is not an approach to be considered in isolation but as part of a multi-disciplinary regime. Each discipline has unique core skills to bring to the assessment of the individual. Each will have expert interventions to offer.

Definitions

Clinically, the term **personality disorder** is preferred to 'psychopath'. Personality disorder has been defined as:

> An enduring pattern of inner experience and behaviour that deviates markedly from the expectations of the individual's culture, is pervasive and inflexible, has an onset in adolescence or early adulthood, is stable over time, and leads to stress or impairment (American Psychiatric Association 2000 p.685)

Both the *Diagnostic and Statistical Manual* (DSM IVR) (American Psychiatric Association 2000) and the *International Classification of Disease* (ICD-10) (World Health Organization 1992) cite a range of personality disorders. However, arguments abound about the labelling of deviant behaviour and whether personality disorder is no more than the medicalization of antisocial behaviour as a means of social control (Porter 1998, Pilgrim and Rogers 1999).

The White Papers outlining the proposed reform of mental health legislation use the term 'those who are dangerous as a result of a severe personality disorder' (Department of Health 2000a, Department of Health 2000b). This is generally interpreted as those with an antisocial personality disorder (American Psychiatric Association 2000) or dissocial personality disorder (World Health Organization 1992) and who present a high risk to society.[1] Critics of the proposal, however, see the scheme as a flawed political gesture that will turn psychiatrists from doctors to jailers (Batty 2002), they believe that a disorder of personality is not amenable to treatment.

Within forensic services there are individuals diagnosed with a range of personality disorders including borderline and histrionic, not just anti-social or dissocial (see Table 20.1 which provides a classification of personality disorders). Additionally, despite advances in international classification, the diagnosis of personality disorders frequently fails to meet tests of reliability and validity (Moran and Hagell 2001). Even the term 'dangerous people with a severe personality disorder' is regarded as a working definition and may be subject to alteration as a clearer picture develops (Department of Health 2000b p.13).

Psychopathic disorder is used here as a legal term. That is, it is one of the four categories of mental disorder (the others being mental illness, mental impairment and severe mental impairment) under which people

---

[1.] These diagnostic categories, although similar, cannot be regarded as identical.

in England and Wales may presently be compulsorily detained in hospital under the Mental Health Act (1983). Within the Act it is defined as:

> A persistent disorder or disability of mind (whether or not including significant impairment of intelligence) which results in abnormally aggressive or seriously irresponsible conduct on the part of the person concerned.
>
> (Mental Health Act 1983 p.2)

A caveat of the Act is that compulsory admission to hospital is permissible only if it 'is likely to alleviate or prevent deterioration of the condition'. Others have used *psychopathy* as a clinical condition and sought instruments to ensure reliable diagnostic assessment (Hare 1991) or have described it as lying at the far end of a spectrum of personality disorders (Prins 1995). But that is not how the term is used here. Instead, psychopathic disorder or psychopathy is considered:

> A legal category describing a number of severe personality disorders which contribute to the person committing anti social acts, usually of a recurrent episodic type.
>
> (Department of Health and Home Office 1994 p.4)

In other words, it is a legal term facilitating admission under the Mental Health Act (1983) and is not used here as a diagnosis. It therefore co-exists with any of the personality disorders in DSM IVR or ICD-10. It can also co-exist with mental illness; so patients may be detained under both categories. Thus, until the Mental Health Act (1983) changes, *psychopathy* is a legal term that does not describe a homogeneous group but is composed of people whose primary diagnosis is not a mental illness.

Diagnosis

The reader is referred to ICD-10 (World Health Organization 1992) and DSM IVR (American Psychiatric Association 2000) for detailed diagnostic criteria both for the general concept of personality disorder and specific personality disorders (see Table 20.1).

These two classifications are similar, and their differences are more related to terminology than content. The development of these categorizations and the different conceptual frameworks that underpin them have been described (Tyrer et al. 1993). For the occupational therapist, one criterion is of particular significance. Personality disorder 'is usually, but not invariably, associated with significant problems in occupational and social performance' (World Health Organization 1992 p.202).

Occupational therapy intervention is based on individual need identified through detailed occupational assessment; therefore diagnostic classification is not an imperative. However, as Dolan and Coid (1993) highlight, a clear diagnosis is essential for research into treatment outcomes.

Table 20.1 Classification of personality disorders

ICD-10	DSM-IVR
F60.0 paranoid personality disorder	301.0 paranoid personality disorder
F60.1 schizoid personality disorder	301.2 schizoid personality disorder
F60.2 dissocial personality disorder	301.7 antisocial personality disorder
F60.3 emotionally unstable personality disorder (.30 impulsive, .31 borderline)	301.83 borderline personality disorder
F60.4 histrionic personality disorder	301.50 histrionic personality disorder
F60.5 anankastic personality disorder	
F60.6 anxious (avoidant) personality disorder	301.82 avoidant personality disorder
F60.7 dependent personality disorder	301.6 dependent personality disorder
	301.22 schizotypal personality disorder
	301.81 narcissistic personality disorder
	301.4 obsessive compulsive disorder
F60.8 other specific personality disorders	
F60.9 personality disorder, unspecified	301.9 personality disorder not otherwise specified

Causal factors

Personality disorders highlight the nature-versus-nurture controversy. Evidence into causation is poor and is sometimes related to criminal behaviour rather than personality disorder. Once all other possible explanations for the disturbed inner experience and behaviour have been excluded, one is left with genetic and environmental influences. Readers wishing to consider the evidence are directed to reviews of risk and causal factors of antisocial and psychopathic personality disorders (Coid 1993, Prins 1995, Moran and Hagell 2001).

Personal experience though suggests that most detained psychopaths have a disrupted and often deprived childhood. There are frequent accounts of early attachments not established or broken, narratives of intermittent institutional care and an environment both emotionally and occupationally deprived. However, not all people with such a history become personality disordered. Nor is it clear what genetic factors may predispose to this history.

Amy's history provides a typical example. Amy is an only child. Both her parents went to prison when she was 13 months old. She was taken into care and returned to her mother's care some six years later. Social Service reports at the time described her mother as inadequate, and several times temporary foster care was arranged. Her mother remarried, and her stepfather, a military man, took over the discipline of Amy. It became a rigid and cruel regime. By her teens, Amy became harder to manage. At school, she defied all authority. Finally, she was placed in a residential unit for maladjusted children. The unit was later criticized for inappropriate use of medication and pin-down policies. There, Amy was involved in several violent incidents. She also had many episodes of self-harm, particularly head banging, cutting and overdoses.

Treatability

A better understanding of causal issues would help support the frames of reference that underpin treatment. For example, in Amy's case how much was learnt by social modelling or acquired as an ego defence mechanism? Was she genetically predisposed to a disorder of personality? Blackburn (1993), who sees personality disorder as learned dysfunctional behaviour, suggests personal 'change' rather than 'cure' should be the goal of treatment with the provision of specific coping skills the most attainable target of intervention.

The proposed new legislation has largely arisen from the conflict surrounding treatability. The present narrow interpretation of treatability, combined with a lack of dedicated provision, has discouraged psychiatrists in all but special hospitals from accepting people deemed psychopathic as detained in-patients (Department of Health and Home Office 1994, Pilgrim and Rogers 1999). In March 2000, in England, 29% of patients in high-security psychiatric hospitals were held under the category of psychopathic disorder. For other NHS facilities, only 2% of detained patients were deemed psychopathic (Department of Health 2000c).

The White Papers signal a clear intent to increase public safety. This is to be accompanied by dedicated services within both prison and health services for people with a severe personality disorder. The first step has been to establish pilot projects providing diagnostic screening and assessment (Home Office 2000, Batty 2002). These endeavours follow a comprehensive review of the research literature that concluded there was insufficient evidence to determine whether personality disorder could be successfully treated (Dolan and Coid 1993). This reviewed physical and pharmacological treatments, psychotherapy (both group and individual), cognitive behavioural therapy, therapeutic communities and long-term-admission milieu therapy. Occupational therapy is cited briefly as one possible ingredient of milieu therapy. The content of the treatment, that is the activities undertaken in the milieu, is not described.

The lack of importance or attention given to the actual treatment received by patients makes commenting about efficacy of specific treatment methods impossible.

(Dolan and Coid 1993 p.205)

Thus, studies could not be measured in terms of efficacy of treatment, but as outcomes of discharge decisions.

Occupational therapy is the profession that considers the therapeutic potential of how individuals spend their time. Therefore, therapists must ensure the contribution of occupational therapy is at least recorded. Outcome measures that isolate the contribution of occupational therapy are notoriously difficult to establish, but as an absolute minimum the aims, objectives and methods of intervention should be recorded and evaluated.

Signs and symptoms

People detained as psychopathic are described as callous individuals lacking any capacity for empathy. They are seen as being grossly irresponsible and as having a very low tolerance to frustration and a low threshold for the discharge of aggression (World Health Organization 1992). Drawing from experience, there are significant features, regardless of the specific personality disorder, that are essential to understand before therapeutic work can begin. These are:

- an aptitude for violence and terror
- power, control and manipulation
- distortion of, or inability to form, relationships
- splitting or fragmentation.

Violence and terror are often the behaviours that determine the person's detention. Sometimes, particularly in women, it is manifested in self-harming behaviour. Frequently, it is directed at others. It is easy to think of the cruel and sadistic crimes that hit the headlines but many are detained with less notoriety. Burt, for example, was admitted to a medium secure unit following repeated verbal and actual assaults on his neighbour. Despite several short custodial sentences, on the day of release from prison he would return to her house. The police had to provide surveillance and protection procedures for her. Aggression is not always expressed directly in violence but conveyed subtly in a sense of latent hostility. For example, in the unit, residents vacated the television lounge when Burt entered. No one challenged him about which programme to watch. Those working with people detained as psychopaths will recognize the occasional days when no incident has occurred; yet there is a real sense of menace, a sense of the potential for terror.

Power, control and manipulation are important facets to recognize. Celia was transferred to a medium secure unit following several years in high security. In many ways, she was lively and popular although she exerted considerable control. Other residents would be both charmed and managed by her. They would fall into a pattern of doing her bidding. At community meetings she would preside, confident she would not be confronted. In more revealing moments she would talk of her 'cherries', the members of staff that she knew she could manipulate. This manipulation can happen almost imperceptibly. Good supervision, allowing introspection and self-reflection, is possibly the best strategy to help the individual worker recognize where their boundaries may have lapsed, for example staying after the shift had ended or becoming engaged in maintaining a secret.

Some psychopaths appear terrified by their sense of power and omnipotence and, seeking external control, behave in such a way as to ensure their detention. After discharge, when Amy was being managed in the community, the situation began to break down. She was made redundant at work and, during an outpatient appointment, she made clear threats to kill her partner and commit suicide. Having established the risk was high, she was invited to return as a voluntary patient. Her admission to the unit, which in one voice she was expressly requesting, was in a violent and hostile manner, with Amy sectioned, handcuffed and under police escort.

Prisoners or patients deemed to have a personality disorder frequently experience **difficulty in relationships**. Some appear unable to form sustained emotional relationships. They may establish relationships but cannot, or do not, develop these to become enduring and emotionally rewarding. For example, despite his accounts of having many friends, Burt never received visitors when he was in the unit. It appeared his social life revolved around alcohol abuse and superficial relationships established at the pub bar. On the other hand, Dominic was admitted to the unit following an attack on his mother. Over the course of time, it was apparent that he had never been able to sustain the warm, intimate relationship which he craved. In a therapeutic moment, he described the continual searching for that one perfect symbiotic relationship. He was able to establish relationships, but, if they began to meet his longing for intimacy he would sabotage or destroy the relationship. Responding to the longing meant, for him, having to relinquish his sense of power and control.

Theories of **splitting or fragmentation**, described in psychoanalytic literature (Cooper 1996) can be directly experienced. It is as though the individual cannot share himself/herself totally with one person. Rather, each person in the team hears and responds to a facet of the person. In some sense, everybody does this, but it is the extent, or degree, to which it occurs in psychopathy that is so stunning. Over the course of my experience, I felt the diagnosis of personality disorder could be predicated on the discord the resident engendered in the team. For example, team discussions about Dominic vacillated between transfer to high security versus unsupervised discharge to the community. Each person was drawing on their own expert, differing and incomplete knowledge of Dominic.

Occupational therapy

A person with a personality disorder, whether in hospital or prison, will not be idle. They have an occupational nature, although the outlet for this may be severely curtailed, restricted or managed. There is neither evidence nor literature to validate the effectiveness of occupational therapy in the treatment of personality disorder, but it is argued that occupational therapy has core skills valuable to any treatment regime. All units, with or without occupational therapists, have intuitively developed some form of activity programme. Indeed, the special hospitals were developed on work ethic principles. Engaging people with personality disorder in activity, however, is often used as a way to manage behaviour, not as a way to address behaviour. There is a very real tension about how violent, manipulative people can be managed to ensure both safety and security. Therefore, fitting people into a regime that manages and contains their antisocial behaviour is understandable, but it is important to establish that being busy, being engaged in activity, is not in itself therapeutic.

Clarity about the core beliefs of occupational therapy helps to explain the different ethos of the occupational therapist to other members of the team. It is a belief in the intrinsic value of activity and occupation, that the drive to act is a basic human need and that engaging in activity can positively influence an individual's health. 'So we exploit this in therapy' (Finlay 1997 p.18). It is about understanding the meaning of occupation to an individual. For people with a personality disorder, their experience of mastery or flow may be intricately bound to antisocial activity. Dominic could move from low self-esteem, not wanting others to see his inadequacy, to feeling powerful and, in a perverse way, respected, when throwing chairs in an angry outburst. It would be naïve to assume acceptable activity can be easily substituted, but striving to find activity where the person can experience autonomy, accomplishment and achievement must have potential. It is also about the balance of occupation and matching appropriately graded activity to identified need. Someone learning skills to cope in a bedsit needs rehearsal and built-in success with every variation of beans on toast, rather than experience the anxiety of expected failure cooking chicken curry.

During my time at Ashen Hill, the model Adaptation through Occupation was used (Reed and Sanderson 1992). The model proved to be both useful and workable in the forensic service. It helped to integrate concepts and provided appropriate schema to encourage consistent assessment that encompassed the diversity of the whole patient group, including those detained as psychopaths. It assisted the analysis of occupational performance and provided a coherent framework to record this. Unlike the Model of Human Occupation, it has not spawned its own assessment tools nor does it guide treatment. This allows an eclectic approach. That is, the model organizes conceptual thinking, but it leaves the therapist to draw on broader frames of reference in treatment planning.

This was particularly useful in the early days at Ashen Hill where, within the limits of a secure environment, a therapeutic community was emulated. For example, the principles of communalism and democratization (Rapoport 1960, Cullen et al. 1997, Jones 2000) can be incorporated into occupational therapy in activities where staff and patients work equally together. Thus writing an admissions leaflet for future residents, preparing and eating a group meal or planning the activity programme became important aspects of the occupational therapy programme. Other settings may draw more on psychodynamic (Cox 1978, Stowell-Smith 2000) or cognitive approaches (Beck et al. 1990). The model of care will not always be a rehabilitative one for there are some people detained as psychopathic who are unlikely ever to leave institutional care. For them, attention is to a quality of life within the institution rather than to a return to the community.

Compounding the symptoms of personality disorder is the anger engendered by compulsory detainment. Added to this there is usually a long history of mistrust, especially of those in a position of authority. It can be a slow and difficult process to build a therapeutic relationship. Building rapport with Celia was not done in an interview. She was suspicious of interviews and, over the years, had completed many checklists and inventories, but she did come to pottery. In pottery, there is a triad of patient, therapist and activity. Indeed, it is this triad that is so valuable when working with people who have a personality disorder. For some patients, a dyadic relationship, for example in individual psychotherapy, is too intense. Much less oppressive is the unstructured group, the chance to engage in something diverting. But the occupational therapist will appreciate the need to use this time to develop trust and understanding. For Celia this was achieved through the vehicle of creative activities.

In the model Adaptation through Occupation, the assessment includes analysis of occupational performance areas, performance skills and the environment. There are three performance areas: self-care, productivity and leisure. It can be conceptually useful to recognize that burglary or drug dealing may be productivity. Balance of occupation is about the interplay of these three areas. Patients returning from high secure hospitals often attend activities by instruction rather than choice. When compulsion is removed, professed leisure pursuits may cease. Adherence to the model helps the therapist discover if this is because the activity reflected mere compliance (productivity) rather than genuine interest (leisure). In the transition from secure setting to community this concept of performance areas directs the therapist's thinking to what is realistically available and how balance in the performance areas may be achieved. For Burt, who was approaching retirement age, the loss of his job was a factor in his index offence. This was recognized and became part of both his treatment and discharge planning. Open employment, given his age and periodic bouts of drinking, was unrealistic, but sheltered employment, begun in the hospital and continued on discharge, helped to structure his week and provide some social contact.

Reed and Sanderson (1983) list five performance skills: motor, sensory, cognitive, intrapersonal and interpersonal skills. Later editions of the model truncate these to three skills, but understanding these five areas, especially separating interpersonal (social relationship) skills and intrapersonal skills (linked, for example, to identity, self-worth and locus of control), is helpful. It is in the analysis of these that many of the disparate problems of personality disorder can be identified. Some people have deficits in every skill component but, with personality disorder, deficits tend to be in the cognitive, intra- and interpersonal domains. In workshop activities, Burt's task ability was good but he worked alongside others, not cooperatively with them. Observation of his occupational performance was revealing good cognitive skills but poorly developed interpersonal skills; whereas, beneath Dominic's façade of confidence were intense feelings of rejection and low self-worth. These intrapersonal deficits were closely allied to his strategies of creating and sabotaging relationships.

Environmental assessment, which includes physical and sociocultural aspects, needs to consider three settings. These are pre-admission, within the unit and proposed future placement. The pre-admission environment for Dominic was homelessness, with some interrupted experience of living in squats. Not until this admission had he practised the skills necessary to live in a bedsit. Eddie was admitted from what he perceived as a brutalizing and victimizing prison regime. Identifying and acknowledging with him how he adapted to prison life provided the first steps in motivating him to acquire alternative skills for future environments.

Activity is the medium for intervention. Although many occupational therapists are undertaking psychodynamic or cognitive group work alongside other professional colleagues, the value of traditional activity must not be underestimated. It can be used in a multitude of ways. At Ashen Hill, thought was given to providing acceptable strategies for managing anger, like wedging clay or heavy digging. For Eddie it was hard and exhausting games of football. Eddie also participated in art therapy, facilitated by an art therapist and occupational therapist. The images on the page became the interface for disclosure. Talking about his drawings revealed how he had idealized his marriage. This idealization compensated for an emotionally arid childhood. However, it could not withstand his wife's infidelity and her hostile denigration of their marriage. These were key issues, leading to him killing her, which were drawn into language through images on the page.

Occupational therapy has much to offer in the treatment of personality disorder, but it is specialized and difficult work. Therefore, occupational therapists need to build on their basic core skills. This can be achieved through reflection on the process, enhanced psychotherapeutic skills and developing self-awareness. To this end, an absolute essential is systematically organized, quality supervision. It is so important it should not be at the mercy of ad hoc arrangements but given time and depth. Occupational therapists can and should extend their psychotherapeutic skills, especially in group work and counselling skills. Depending on the ethos of the setting, advanced psychodynamic or cognitive skills will be beneficial. Finally, the deeper the self-understanding the therapist has, the deeper the level of work that can be undertaken. I would therefore argue that all staff wishing to work therapeutically with people who have a personality disorder should undertake an extended period of their own personal therapy.

Conclusion

At present, there is no evidence for the efficacy of occupational therapy for people diagnosed as having a personality disorder despite many having significant impairment in occupational and social performance. Future researchers, hopefully, will establish empirical evidence for what is put forward here. That is, despite the controversy surrounding this group of individuals, occupational therapy can change the tasks engaged in from diversion or management strategies to effective therapeutic intervention. Within a multidisciplinary team, occupational therapists have complementary skills valuable to both hospital and prison settings. The difficult nature of working with personality disordered people is acknowledged, and skill development and good supervision are necessary. Additionally, occupational therapists need to communicate better what it is they do both in their dialogue with the team and in patients' notes so that outcomes can be measured.

References

American Psychiatric Association (2000) Diagnostic and Statistical Manual of Mental Disorders (4th edition) (DSM IVR). Washington DC: American Psychiatric Association.

Batty D (2002) Risky View. The Guardian. London: Downloaded from http://society.guardian.co.uk on 19 April 2002.

Beck A and Freeman A (1990) Cognitive Therapy of Personality Disorders. New York: The Guilford Press.

Blackburn R (1993) Clinical programmes with psychopaths. In: Clinical Approaches to the Mentally Disordered Offender, Howells K and Hollis C (eds.) Chichester: John Wiley.

Coid J (1993) Current concepts and classifications of psychopathic disorder. In: Personality Disorder Reviewed, Tyrer P and Stein G (eds.). London: The Royal College of Psychiatrists/Gaskell.

Cooper C (1996) Psychodynamic therapy: The Kleinian approach. In: Handbook of Individual Therapy, Dryden W (ed.). London: Sage Publications.

Cox M (1978) Structuring the Therapeutic Process: Compromise with Chaos. Oxford: Pergamon Press.

Cullen E, Jones L and Woodward R (eds.) (1997) Therapeutic Communities for Offenders. Wiley Series in Offender Rehabilitation. Chichester: John Wiley and Sons.

Department of Health (2000a) Reforming the Mental Health Act: (Part I) The New Legal Framework. London: The Stationery Office.

Department of Health (2000b) Reforming the Mental Health Act: (Part II) High-risk Patients. London: The Stationery Office.

Department of Health (2000c) Inpatients Formally Detained in Hospitals under the Mental Health Act 1983 and Other Legislation, England: 1989–1990 to 1999–2000. London: Department of Health.

Department of Health and Home Office (1994) Report of the Department of Health and Home Office Working Group on Psychopathic Disorder, chaired by Dr J Reed. London: Department of Health and Home Office.

Dolan B and Coid J (1993) Psychopathic and Antisocial Personality Disorders: Treatment and Research Issues. London: Gaskell.

Finlay L (1997) The Practice of Psychosocial Occupational Therapy. Cheltenham: Stanley Thornes.

Hare R (1991) Manual for the Hare Psychopathy Checklist – Revised. Toronto: Multi-health Systems.

Home Office (2000) Pilot Project to Assess Dangerous Severe Personality Disorder Announced by Home Office. London: http://www.homeoffice.gov.uk, downloaded 22 February 2000.

Jones L (2000) Therapeutic community in a forensic setting. In: Forensic Mental Health Care: A Case Study Approach, Mercer D, Mason T, McKeown M and McCann G (eds.). Edinburgh: Churchill Livingstone.

Moran P and Hagell A (2001) Intervening to Prevent Antisocial Personality Disorder: A scoping review. London: Home Office Research, Development and Statistical Directorate.

Pilgrim D and Rogers A (1999) A Sociology of Mental Illness. Buckingham: Open University Press.

Porter S (1998) The social interpretation of deviance. In: Sociology as Applied to Nursing and Health Care, Birchenall M and Birchenall P (eds.). London: Baillière Tindall.

Prins H (1995) Offenders, Deviants or Patients? London: Routledge.

Rapoport R (1960) The Community As Doctor. London: Tavistock Publications.

Reed K and Sanderson S (1983) Concepts of Occupational Therapy. Baltimore: Williams and Wilkins.

Reed K and Sanderson S (1992) Concepts of Occupational Therapy (3rd edition). Baltimore: Williams and Wilkins.

Stowell-Smith M (2000) Psychodynamic psychotherapy, personality disorder and offending. In: Forensic Mental Health Care: A Case Study Approach, Mercer D, Mason T, McKeown M and McCann G (eds.). Edinburgh: Churchill Livingstone.

Tyrer P, Casey P and Ferguson B (1993) Personality disorder in perspective. In: Personality Disorder Reviewed, Tyrer P and Stein G (eds.). London: Gaskell.

World Health Organization (1992) The ICD-10 Classification of Mental and Behavioural Disorders: Clinical descriptions and diagnostic guidelines. Geneva: World Health Organization.

Index

OT stands for Occupational Therapy

Printed in the United Kingdom
by Lightning Source UK Ltd.
116628UKS00001B/121-147